Happy Gerson

Recipes & Tips to Make Healing Fun

Helen Bairstow & Others

Dedicated to all the angels on earth…

Contents

Foreword by Howard Straus, grandson of Dr Max Gerson...

Having lived and worked around the Gerson Therapy all my life due to my mother being Dr. Gerson's daughter, I have built up a gradual but complete acceptance of the effectiveness of the Therapy against all manner of "chronic" or "degenerative" illnesses, from the annoying but relatively benign migraine to advanced, "terminal" cancers, including melanoma, pancreatic cancer and lymphoma. I have administered the Therapy as a clinic administrator, clinic founder, patient, husband of a cancer recovery. I have watched patients with dozens of different "incurable" ailments recover and reclaim their health, return to their lives, and improve the overall health of their families and entire communities. And, inevitably, there are some patients who don't recover; after all, allopathic medicine has given up virtually all Gerson patients as "terminal" before they even think of coming to this stringent, work-intensive, lifestyle-altering therapy. Of the patients who choose other approaches, most shun the treatment simply because of the extreme change in their prospective lifestyle. Others reject the idea of the coffee enema as "too radical". (Interesting, since they do not hesitate to have small or large, peripheral or important organs removed and discarded!) Many cannot afford, or cannot obtain in their locality the required organic foods necessary to the execution of the Therapy, others use the relative unavailability as an excuse not to have to change their food choices. We wish them well with their choices.

But there is a steady, and increasing number of people who have heard of the successes of the Therapy from friends, recovered patients, often from one of the several Gerson documentaries produced by master film-maker Steve Kroschel of Haines, AK, or snippets of documentaries made by many others that include cuts of Charlotte Gerson and/or recovered Gerson patients, alive 5, 10, 30, even 50 years after their predicted demise by conventional physicians! These are inspiring, heroic stories of snatching life from the very jaws of "certain" death that cannot help but move at least some to strike out in a very different direction than the acceptable and generally disastrous results produced by today's conventional medical practice.

These outliers are our heroes, people who have stared the "beast" in the eye from inches away, and made it back down. I applaud them. The people who read this book have already made an awesome decision, and that is to reject the standard wisdom of every doctor and medical expert they know, and often their own families' entreaties, and do something very different, with a century-long record of success in restoring health to the most desperate of patients.

Happy Gerson is written to encourage and bolster the commitment of those who face the daunting physical and psychological barriers to success in implementing the Gerson Therapy. They have seen the seemingly insurmountable and endless list of tasks to be accomplished, the almost complete change in their eating habits, the apparently bizarre routine of multiple daily coffee enemas, the long list of "forbidden" foods, and almost despaired. They have often started their journeys at a Gerson Therapy clinic, under the care of an experienced Gerson Therapy practitioner, and have no idea how they will manage to implement it all when they return to their homes. Yet, the thousands, dare I say tens of thousands of success stories of "miraculous" recoveries show that this is a regime that, strange and different as it may seem at the beginning, will yield rapid and stunning results that generally do more to encourage the persistent patient than to discourage him/her. After some initial months of the shock of change, it all becomes rather routine, tastes change, results begin to appear, and it all becomes more of the "new normal" of the patient's life.

Ms. Bairstow has addressed the numerous departures from normal life that this therapy entails, and put a human face on them. She writes with a humor and humanity that accepts exhaustion, discouragement, familial disruption, and says, "Okay, today was not a perfect day, but tomorrow, we start all over again, with a clean slate and another opportunity to do it better." Along the way, she has put together a really good list of tasty Gerson-compliant recipes (including beautiful photographs) that made my mouth water and made me wish I could sit down to such a meal. Other patients have helped her along the way, contributing their experiences, successes and, yes, disappointments and failures, recipes and comical incidents (like carrot pulp on the ceiling), necessities and hints to make it all easier. Happy Gerson is a guidebook and journey map for the Gerson newbie. It is not a substitute for the Therapy book, any more than a cheerleading team will win a football game. But cheerleaders encourage the crowd, the players, and help the team to come away with a win, if possible.

So, for all you Gerson "freshmen" out there, know that you are not the only one who has gone through the fire. You are not the first one to have doubts, fears and hurdles. Many others have done so, many have succeeded, and they are willing to help you, to be your cheerleaders. But you are ultimately the one who must implement this lifesaving and restorative therapy on your own. You have company aplenty, those who have gone before, those who are just starting. Welcome to the first day of the rest of your lives!

Howard Straus, Carmel, CA

Chapter 1: What To Expect From This Book (and what <u>NOT</u> to expect)

"The soil is our external metabolism. It must be free of herbicides and pesticides or the body cannot heal."
Dr. Max Gerson

Hello! Thank you for purchasing this book knowing that all proceeds go to Gerson Therapy charities.

This is a book for peeps like us who are undertaking the Gerson Therapy. We call ourselves "Gerson Persons". Even though it says it is written (or rather 'put' together) by me, Helen Bairstow, so many other Gerson Persons have contributed to make this book possible. Thanks guys. I started full time Gerson Therapy in 2014 to heal stage four breast cancer and this book is a way for me to share my journey, and … lots of recipes.

My wish is for this book to help make *"Happy"* Gerson persons (and raise money).

Enjoy.
Helen

This Book May <u>NOT</u> Be For You

If you want to find out about the Gerson Therapy, this book is not for you.

The best book for learning all about and how to do the Gerson Therapy is "Healing the Gerson Way" by Charlotte Gerson, daughter of Dr Max

Gerson, ("Healing the Gerson Way", available from the Gerson Institute www.gerson.org and also on Amazon).

Happy Gerson is *absolutely* not a replacement for any Gerson Institute information. This book has been written for people who already 'know' about the Gerson Therapy and have even started the protocol. It will also be a good read for those supporting a loved one on the therapy who maybe want to get a bit of an understanding of what it is like to be on the therapy. If you are on the therapy or a support person, either way, you will be pleased to know everything you read here is purely following the principles laid down by Dr Max Gerson ... **every word is Gerson "friendly"**.

Data overload can be experienced when starting, or considering, the Gerson Therapy so this book has been written 'lightly' with snippets of humor and humanness, designed to read cover to cover or, to be picked up when needing a bit of inspiration or a recipe to entice a lagging appetite.

Right Words At The Right Time

When contemplating if this book 'needed' to be written, I received this message from a fellow Gerson Person... *"There is a special unmatchable gift that comes from knowing you are not alone... from sharing our experiences and coming along side one-another in our journeys... lifting each other up, validating feelings, and sorting out pieces in the puzzle that is our own very personal healing process... it's such a raw, honest, beautiful thing - absolutely so thankful for those who have shared and continue to share - it's a different, very unique, kind of friendship and it's priceless. Thanks so much for caring enough about so many to bravely share from your own journey. Pouring yourself out into so many - beautiful, Helen, beautiful... time well spent."* So thank you *Rae Stroud* for the right words at the right time to give me the encouragement to publish this.

Making A Difference…Together

All proceeds go to two Gerson Therapy charities.

1. The Carrot Fund (www.thecarrotfund.com). The Carrot Fund is a charity set up to raise money for people doing The Gerson Therapy who are having financial difficulties and can use assistance in purchasing their Gerson supplements.
2. The Gerson Institute (www.gerson.org), a not-for-profit organization that tirelessly works to make Gerson Therapy information readily available to the public.

So … here's to sharing the Gerson Therapy, love and laughter…

A Day in the Gerson Therapy Life of a Gerson Person … Me!

I put this on my Facebook page one day and my friends were so surprised to actually see in real time everything involved. So…if you're reading this as a support person, or thinking of beginning the protocol, it might give you a small insight of what's involved.

8 am:

First juice is my favourite! Orange. Or even better … grapefruit! And… one litre (2 pints) of coffee!

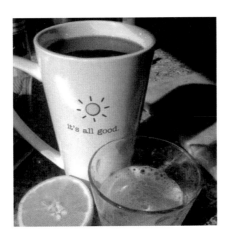

Breakfast:

Slow cooked organic oats with a piece of poached unsulphured organic dried fruit, non fat yogurt, flaxseed oil and a tad of honey!

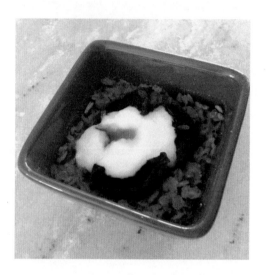

9 am:

Green juice. This is what's in it today!

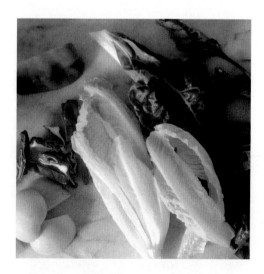

The official Gerson Green Juice

1 small wedge red cabbage

1/4 green bell pepper/capsicum

1 leaf endive

1 leaf chard/silverbeet

2 leaves beet tops (inner small leaves)

2 sprigs watercress

1 large handful of cos, green or red leaf lettuce (not iceberg)

1 medium green apple, cored (seeds removed)

IMPORTANT: Do not substitute for green vegetables that you may not be able to get. (*Some days my green juice has been apple and lettuce.*)

10 am:

Carrot and apple juice. Clean the juicer…again.

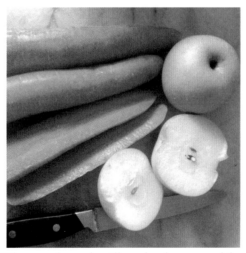

(Of course the seeds will need to be removed first.)

11 am:

What time is it? It's juice time! Bugger using a glass. Just more washing up and no one's watching…

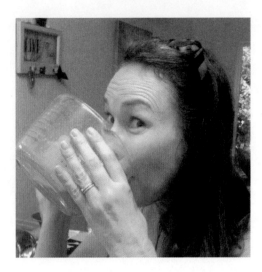

12 noon(ish):
Running late (nothing new) with fifth juice of the day, carrot and apple.

12.30pm:
Coffee time! Another litre bites the dust! Milly is my coffee buddy. Washed and prepared the potatoes which are cooking in oven for lunch while I have coffee.

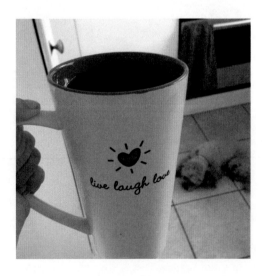

Lunch 1pm(ish):

Zucchini pasta with blended raw corn, celery and honey/flax oil/lemon juice (yes, recipe will be in recipe section!). With potatoes (that I put in oven before coffee) and non-fat yogurt. And Hippocrates soup.

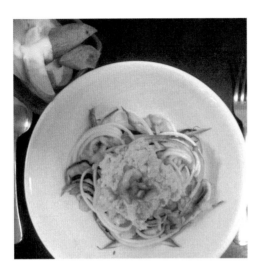

2pm:

Typical… having my 1pm juice at 2pm. This is a good day! And … it's time to clean the juicer!

2.30pm:

Juice seven for the day! Phew when I make it to this one I can relax a little. Next juice not until 4! This gives me a window to pick up my son from school or go out. (I'm on the Modified Gerson Therapy of 10 juices and 3 coffees often referred to as 10/3. The full protocol is 13/5. I am in awe of those doing the full Gerson Therapy.)

4pm:

Apple and carrot time! And … clean the juicer!

5pm:

Coffee time! Yep, another litre. If you haven't worked it out by now, I'm

NOT drinking it but I'm definitely not taking a picture of that!

6pm:

Second to last juice for the day. Carrot or green? You guess which one? Side Effects Warning: clown around syndrome and desire to enter the 'who can raise their eyebrows the highest' competition! (You'll read further evidence later how important it is to have a sense of humor doing this therapy!)

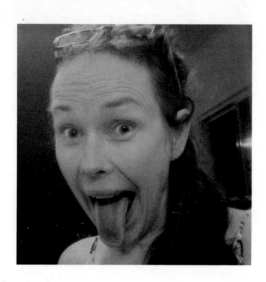

Dinner:

Baked potato topped with stuff and a yogurt mint cilantro sauce. Plus a mug of the special Hippocrates soup. And not over yet ... there's still one more juice to go...

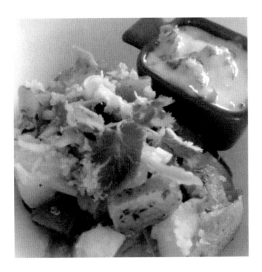

8pm:

Ta da! I did it. Last juice. That's 10! And my reward (apart from healing my body!) is... I get to do it all again tomorrow! When asked what's the one thing I miss? My answer is being hungry! Look at everything I eat *every* day! So... hungry? Never!

So 'why' did I record a day in my life? Fun. Maybe. What I've learned is that I can DO it by myself, without help, but I couldn't keep it up. Energy is a premium commodity for anyone doing Gerson as your body needs the energy to 'renovate and repair'. And there wasn't much rest today. Simply put, the Gerson Therapy works by the organic juices and food supplying continuous nutrition and the 'coffee' gets the rubbish out via the liver. What I DIDN'T do today ... any house work or laundry, prepare the coffee concentrate, watch TV, have a 'nanna nap', play 'Words with Friends', go anywhere! ... I didn't even have a shower! So tomorrow I'm welcoming back my 'angels' who help me because having help is not a luxury it is a necessity.

Chapter 2: If Only I Knew! Emotions, Stalling Tactics and Funny Stories

"When you cannot accept and ask for help without self-judgement, then when you offer other people help you are doing so with judgement."
Dr Rene Brown

Gerson Life

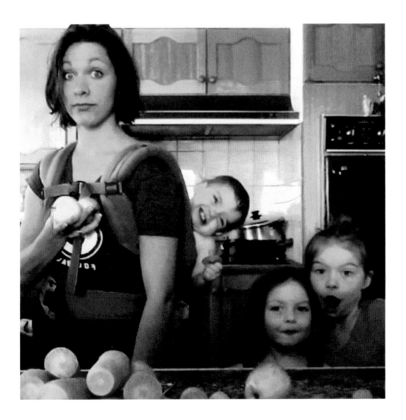

This photo absolutely depicts life on Gerson. The chaos, the never ending produce and jobs, the laughter, the essential silliness, the healing love, our ability to ask for help and to do what has to be done, in whatever way necessary. Thanks Rachel Sharman for sharing. On Rachel's back is Violet, then Norah is next and Eva is the eldest on the right.

Why Don't We Think We Deserve To Get Help?

I think that for women who may have seen our mothers keep a clean tidy house (or the opposite) there's a part of us that finds getting 'help' to house clean a failure. But it's not. It's smart. We cannot heal if we are exhausted from cleaning. And if a clean tidy organised household aides your healing then you need that too. Just let someone else do it, someone who may need that money or purpose.

An African proverb says "It takes a village to raise a child." I say "It takes a team of 'angels' to do Gerson Therapy."

Get Help…Ask For Angels

Get help for chores, especially for chores that you don't like. Split chores up so your angels all get a go. For example … someone could make Hippocrates soup twice a week. They can do this at home and then drop it off. Another angel could make salad or Gerson recipe and drop it off. Another could clean house once a week. Shopping or picking up organic orders can help too. Perhaps your partner could make the first one or two juices before going to work and store them in a thermos to keep them fresher, but apple and carrot juice only, as the green juice must be drunk immediately because it oxidizes faster.

Funny Stories But... Only Gerson Therapy Peeps May Find These Funny

<u>WARNING</u>: If you're yet to do coffee enemas (CE) DON'T read these stories. If you've chalked up many coffees then you may get a laugh, or a knowing smile at least!

~~~~ ~~~~

"Many times I've thought about painting bathroom walls (and ceiling) dark brown to save the inevitable!" *Helen Bairstow*

~~~~ ~~~~

"Yesterday was my FIRST time with the CE so I thought I would share my experience. Well... Ummm... Ok... My yoga mat needs to be burned, my floor, walls, toilet and tub all need to be professionally cleaned, my shower has never seen that kind of mess and I don't think I have laughed this hard for a really long time! In fact I haven't stopped laughing since yesterday! Round two here I go!! Ha!" *Sherry Sweet*

~~~~ ~~~~

"Oh you'll get the strangest responses and comments from people when they learn what the Gerson Therapy entails... a well meaning person says to me 'I looked up online coffee enemas and you can die from them!' Without missing a beat I replied... 'You can die of cancer too!' She's standing there stunned and looking confused so I continue... 'How many people do you know who have died of cancer?' 'Lots' she says and I finish ... 'How many people do you know who have died of coffee enemas!'" *Helen Bairstow*

~~~~ ~~~~

ROFL Stories From Jfur

You'll get to recognize Jfur's quirky way of telling stories and making light of what weaker people might call disastrous situations! (Oh in case you're wondering, ROFL = Rolling On Floor Laughing)

"I do coffee enemas in the bath tub with an old yoga mat for insulation. You can get pretty good at letting out some of the fluid in the tub if needed (while holding in the chunks), so that when you stand up there's not so much pressure to release. Also, I find there are cycles of 'need to release', and if you can lay still and hold until they pass, then you can make it easier to the toilet. It's a timing thing. However, when there's gas, all bets are off!" *Jfur Simpson*

~~~~ ~~~~

"WARNING: Once you have sat on the toilet to evacuate your CE, DO NOT, I repeat, DO NOT bend over for ANY reason (no matter WHAT may have dropped on the floor). It appears the "ready to be evacuated" Coffee Enema has the force, distance, and coverage of a small hydraulic hose (just sayin'). Good times!" *Jfur Simpson*

~~~~ ~~~~

Gotta laugh at this from *Nicole Mackey* … "I have answered the door to Jehovah Witnesses with a full butt and listened to them during cramps until I say gotta go!"

~~~~ ~~~~

More 'toilet' humor that long term Gerson Persons, unfortunately, understand from *Christina Holly Juarez*'s mom.

"Did you hear about the guy who went to the Dr. for his hemorrhoids?"
"The Dr. prescribed him suppositories, and when he went for his return check up, the Dr. asked, so, how're the suppositories helping?"
Then the guy says "Man! For as awful as they tasted, I coulda shoved them up my a$%!"

Red Faced

"Just got through chatting with my daughter's ballet teacher and had a niacin flush take over right as we started talking. She acted like nothing was happening at first but then a few minutes in she obviously couldn't help herself and said "Um, are you ok?! You are so red. Are you going to pass out?" Haha no, no… just the perks of the therapy my friend." *Rachel Sharman*

Some Days You Feel Like Kicking the Dog!

Here's a post from me in the Facebook Gerson Therapy Support Group, on one of 'those' days…

"Six months in and I was going fine but I'm so emotional. Feeling lonely. Separate from everyone not on Gerson Therapy. Today I just feel like no one understands. Even my husband. Flew off the handle at him tonight when he asked if I wanted my last juice. I refused to have it. Stormed out the kitchen saying I'm so over all this. Just wish it'd all go away. Very unlike me. Yelled at Elliot (my 9 year old son). Not sure what's going on. Hopefully tomorrow's a better day. If I kick the dog I'm committing myself!"

Rae Stroud replied beautifully… "Oh friend you are so very not alone. Wish I could give you a great big (((hug))). Healing is such a strange road… I'm not typically emotional either but boy have I had my moments/days! The more I read, the more I'm comforted with the natural ebb and flow of healing… it's all part of it… the good, the bad, and the ugly! … give yourself Grace friend… look at the road you've come down and give yourself some acknowledgment for how far you've come. And so much love… here's to brand new days, fresh starts, and new beginnings."

Express It My Friends

Leanna Little Prosser "Today is one of those days where I don't want to juice one more carrot…! I actually don't mind drinking it I just don't feel like doing everything involved to produce it. Just thinking how nice it would be if I could just access my port and IV my carrot juice into me with one of those chemo fanny packs. Refill it once a week and call it good! Oh well, no use complaining…I mean I only have two to three years left to go!"

Seeing Things Differently

For me I had to learn a new skill … the ability to NOT see stuff! Learning to ignore jobs that need to be done and rest instead. Sounds easy but it wasn't. I had to learn to love a "lived-in" looking house. Which for me, as a recovering workaholic, was easier said than done, really. I discovered I had to decipher the difference between resting and being lazy.

Look for the Silver Lining

Yes doing Gerson Therapy is hard work but there are many unexpected, and very pleasant, surprises you'll notice. Like…

- Discovering the joy of simplifying life.
- Not watching food television programs. What's the point!
- Buying hardly anything from a regular supermarket.
- Washing up is so easy because there's no oil. Except flaxseed oil. So you use hardly any detergent. You can even use cold water to wash up in.

- The camaraderie of Gerson Therapy support groups. A bit like when you have a baby and find a like minded mothers group.

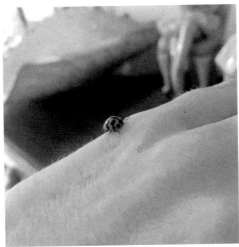

Unexpected 'delightful' surprises ... how's this for proof that you ARE eating organic produce!

There's Wisdom When We Listen

Rene Ready shares a funny story that has wisdom within... "I work in Home Health as a therapist with old people mostly. I love it! Anyways, today an old guy invited me to have lunch with him and his wife. I declined and said I just ate a whole cauliflower with tomato sauce and parsley. He didn't miss a beat and said "You will never get cancer". Too bad more people didn't think like that."

Live Laugh Love

Betsy Geist captured how great you can feel "pro" healing reaction...
"Fever has broooo-ken, like the first morrrrrrrrrn-ing. Blackbird has spoooooo-ken, like the first bird..." A good morning report, feeling massively better today. Thank you for the well-wishes. I'm pretty sure a couple billion cancer cells bit the dust yesterday. Bye-bye. It was nice

knowing ya. NOT.

Leanna Little Prosser reminds us that laughter is good for the body and soul by sharing this hilarious snippet with us…

So I get this text this morning from my sweet husband which spins out of 'Gerson Pun' control. Here's how it went:

Him "Who needs a gerber baby when you have a Gerson baby! Luv u."

Me "Who's a cheeky monkey! Love u!"

Him "I know, I live in a house full of them! If you can't BEET them, join them! (I eat beets twice a day on Gerson)

Me "Beets…was that an intentional pun hun?"

Him "A lame attempt, must be honest, can't be a Hippocrates, have a SOUPER day!"

Me "Good one ha ha!"

Him "So in a flash of inspiration, I have a business idea. We can start a franchise business offering the Gerson coffee break thing, we'll call it STARBUTTS! Lots of flavors too! Well maybe not?! Life's too short to make ENEMAS!"

Me "Bwahahahaha! You've really outdone yourself!"

Him "Starlight, starbright got a tube in my bum tonite!"

Me (after I couldn't resist sharing the fun with my Gerson Team - sister and her husband) "Roger said next time you make a Star Wars convention, you can be JAVA the BUTT!"

Him "I'd rather be HAM SOLO (vegan pun) or maybe R2 DETOX!"

And it was Leanna who also found this appropriate yoga mat to use during coffee time!

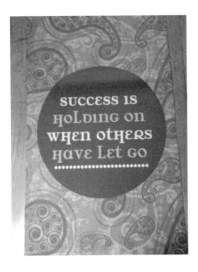

Healing The 'Hard' Stuff

Anonymous has extremely wise lessons for us...

"As part of my emotional healing on Gerson Therapy...I'm traveling today to see my dad in the hospital. He has been drinking himself to death over the last thirty years and he is in the ICU after surgery to repair the ulcers in his esophagus. He collapsed yesterday because of the internal bleeding he has been ignoring yet continues drinking. I've only seen him twice in ten years because I can't/won't tolerate the trail of destruction that follows him and those around him. My younger brother has been guilting me for months saying it's our responsibility to care for him since nobody is left. (Insert all those al-anon statements here). As I pack my new baby up and all the Gerson supplies I will need for this road trip...I'm so angry that I'm fighting for my health and every precious second with my family and children while he chooses to give his up. But I've decided to be the bigger person and if I can bring him some comfort in his final time with us then that's what I'll do and let the rest go for my own health and happiness. I love him and pray he is at peace.

My family (my partner and children) will always come first along with my health! After so many years away from the situation to reflect, it's easier to see it from a more adult perspective. I am blessed to have all the amazing things he has missed out on…a beautiful home, a loving spouse, and all the joy my children bring me each day as I watch them grow. He is a sick old man alone and in pain in a hospital bed …and it's too late to take back the choices he's made. It isn't a place I'd wish on anybody at the end of their time on this earth. There's a difference between sympathy and empathy…I can at least empathize with the situation…I cannot judge whatever happened in his life to lead him down this path since I haven't walked in his shoes. His mother, my grandmother, passed away this last summer. She was the most kind and gentle person I've known and handled everything she went through with Grace and love. I'm going to try to do the same. As for my brother…I understand he is desperate to provide whatever measure of comfort he can to the father he's always hoped to have a relationship with. As the person who has mothered him during his life, I can also empathize with his feelings…even if I don't agree with them… and understand how he could feel let down because I haven't jumped to the rescue in this matter."

3 days later … "Left for home this afternoon…my dad is awake and feeling well enough to insist we smuggle alcohol into his hospital room. When that failed he got my step mom to sneak him opiates to take in conjunction with the doses the hospital is already administering to him. Too much for me to watch…very sad. The doctor this morning gave him a list of support groups to help stop drinking and they have given him drugs to stop withdrawal symptoms when he is released-they told him the next time it's very likely he will bleed to death before the ambulance reaches him. It's so painful to watch my younger siblings get their hopes up that this will be the time it will finally click for him and he will recover. It's a nice hope…I wanted to offer to stay in the guest room for a few weeks and make batches of Hippo soup and Gerson juices for him to help him heal…but didn't. You cannot help somebody that doesn't want help and the enabling is too toxic to be around…I have to care for myself! I'm glad we came to see him and he met his grandchild. The moment we closed the car door in the parking lot all the drama faded away and our family was back in our happy love bubble…so grateful for what I have in my life."

Chapter 3: Intestinal Fortitude - You CAN Do This

"Natural forces within us are the true healers of disease."
Hippocrates

Doing Gerson Therapy has taught me (finally) to let go of perfection (it's totally overrated!) and aim instead for excellence. And … I think the definition of "excellent" is the BEST you can do in that moment!

Just Like … Running A Marathon

You don't wake up one day and decide you're going to run a marathon the next day. You train for it. If you've never run before, 42 kilometres seems unachievable. But running around the block could be achievable! Then 5 kilometres, then 10, building yourself up to the marathon.

Getting ready to do the Gerson Therapy is like preparing for a **two year** marathon. Start at your pace. It took me three months to build up to the full therapy, starting with just three juices and one coffee.

Plus in order to run a marathon you're going to need the right equipment, like good running shoes, and a support team to encourage you during training and hand you water on race day.

How Big Is Your Why

If you've got the choice of dying or doing Gerson Therapy for two years it's a "no-brainer". You CAN do this. Will power becomes obsolete.

Be Easy On Yourself

Some days ... I don't wash the carrots.

Some days ... instead of cleaning juicer between juices I pour hot water in it.

Some days ... I don't even do that between juices.

Some days ... I eat soup before it goes through the Mouli.

Some days ... I don't eat soup!

Some days ... I have to force myself to drink another juice!

Some days ... I don't even shower as I'm too busy doing it all.

Some days ... I 'have' to have five showers!

More Unexpected Outcomes

Another unexpected benefit is the liberating feeling of NOT having other food. Not even THINKING about other food. When you read a magazine, you simply skip food section. When you go to a shopping mall, you skip the food court. When food ads come on TV, you just zone out. When a 'health' report or article is sent, you skip it (unless it's from the Gerson Institute) and even grocery shopping is easier as you just buy your Gerson supplies and don't waste grey matter (or healing energy) on trying or buying new stuff. You get a sense of achievement having made the decision to eat and live this way. Celebrate it.

And who ever thought... you'd actually look FORWARD to coffee enemas!

Notice Your Achievements

Melissa Gravano sure did on this day...

"Prior to today and for a few days I was feeling VERY frustrated with my Gerson journey, coffee breaks especially, and feeling WAY TOO home bound. I had a date with the oncologist today. I wanted to reschedule but my intuition, (and every time I prayed I got a big DO NOT CANCEL). He has been unpleasant at times in the past but this time I wasn't nervous, I just have a lot going on this week is why I was thinking of rescheduling. At the last minute my friend sent her husband to take me instead of her, and her husband turned out to be a pleasant chatterbox, which was good for me to take my mind off of myself.

The drive and scenery was very pleasant and relaxing. The good ole' doc was more diplomatic than usual and he gave me some helpful feedback about my blood work. The thing that amazed me is I managed to do more juicings today, (ten), than I did on Saturday for example when I made myself stay home and not attend a meeting I really wanted to attend, so I could "take care of myself." I never did figure out where that morning went and how it came to be that I didn't start juicing until 2:00 p.m. I also become so wretchedly angry that I cracked my wooden juicing dowel while crying and slamming it in my juicer. I got some relief when I made my carrot juices and took them with me to the woods which is where I needed to be.

I have been ruminating with my mentors about my coffee break issues and after praying got the message that the thing to do is to quit thinking about them and just do them however they come out. I kept writing affirmations and claiming faith in my healing then the next minute fell into fear and doubt about not doing it right. I finally remembered one of my sayings. Do my best and God will do the rest, and it's good enough!

Oh, yea, my visit to the oncologist has a very useful purpose. I could hear him in the other room talking to a patient about chemo. It renewed my sense of gratitude for the gift of Gerson Therapy. When I returned home and ended up with a 2 cup 15 minute enema I was truly peaceful and ok with it. Low and behold, my last enema of the day turned out to be 4 cups and 15 minutes, and with very little struggle!

So this is my bedtime story for all ya'll who might have your teddy bears or like me, your stuffed bunny rabbits in hand, ready to go sleepy. Oh! By the way, I have this on going craving for fried chicken, someone in my home went to bed and left my favorite in a box on the table. A nice juicy crunchy thigh. I smelled it, it was from some chain so it was kind of gross anyway, but if I could have I would have, but I didn't. Sweet dreams!"

Chapter 4: We're In This Together

"Everything that can be counted does not necessarily count; everything that counts cannot necessarily be counted."
Albert Einstein

Be prepared that people, even people close to you, may not understand what it is like to be on the Gerson Therapy but recognize that people love you and want you to succeed.

You may find the only people who *really* understand are others doing the therapy so find yourself a support group that you can join, like the Gerson Therapy Support Group on Facebook. It is a closely monitored closed group. Simply go to Facebook, search for Gerson Therapy Support Group and request to become a member.

Deborah Felton expresses completely what its like to be a member of the Gerson Therapy Support Group … *"I just want to say how grateful I am. Grateful for Gerson Therapy, grateful for the chance to heal and grateful for this group* (Gerson Therapy Support Group on Facebook) *with all of it's beautiful members, recipes, support, resources, friendship and understanding that only you can give. You all mean so very much to me. I don't know if I could do this without you."*

"Essentials" You Might <u>NOT</u> Have Thought Of

I wanted to include in this this book for a list of things you 'have' to have when doing the Gerson Therapy so we asked experienced Gerson persons. There was a surprise list posted from *Jfur Simpson* that was not 'things' but are surprisingly essential.

- Internet connection and Facebook support group
- Gerson 'angels' who help however they can (soup angels, shopping angels)
- Sense of humor (including the ability to laugh at yourself)
- Sense of survival
- Indomitable spirit
- The patience of a saint and the courage of a gladiator
- Someone to laugh about it with
- Persistence
- The ability to fall down seven times and get up eight!
- The ability to multitask or the willingness to learn
- A willingness to learn how to apologize
- A willingness to learn how to ask for what you need
- Nerves of steel and a nose of lilacs
- The willingness to hang in there until the soup becomes enjoyable!

Love On Four Legs

If you have a pet, you'll always have a source of unconditional love. Even when you are lying on the bathroom floor with a tube up your "you know what"!

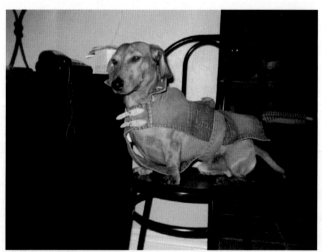

My little Junior was with me from my diagnosis to the end... I don't know what I would have done without him when I was feeling scared. *Doris Parreno*

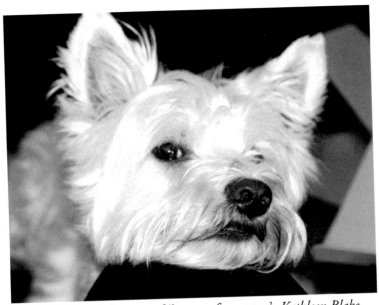

Toby is the definition of 'love on four paws'. *Kathleen Blake*

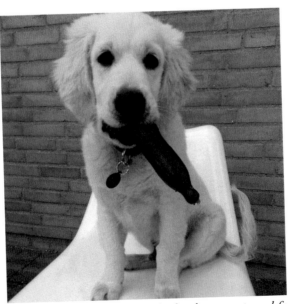

"Well there were no carrots left so I had to have my second favorite!"

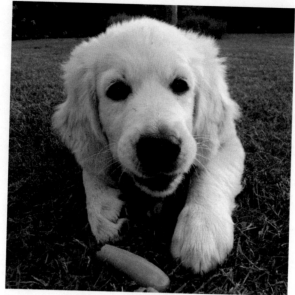

"Look mom I found the carrots!"

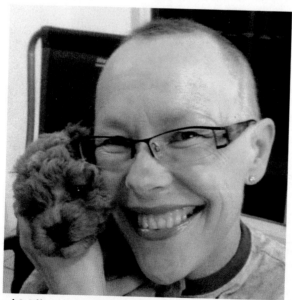

Helen and Milly taken June 2011 (6 months after I was diagnosed) after finishing chemo (which explains the hair style!).

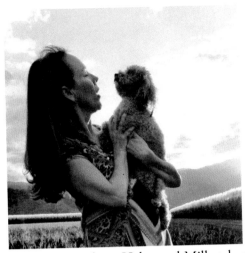

A picture tells a 1000 words … Helen and Milly taken July 2014
(6 months into Gerson Therapy). As Milly grows
into a mature dog I see my survival success.
"I am so privileged to be loved this much by an animal." Helen Bairstow

Rene Ready's Dogs Delight Us All

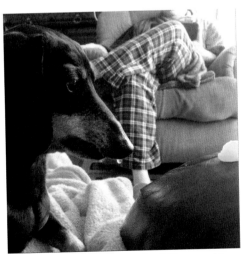

Drooling and slobbering while waited for the OK to eat his orange snack! Super healthy Gerson dog, the vet can't believe he is 11 yrs old.

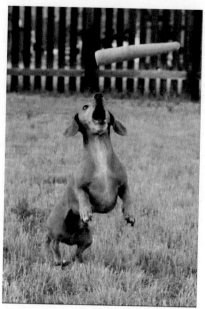

Catch!

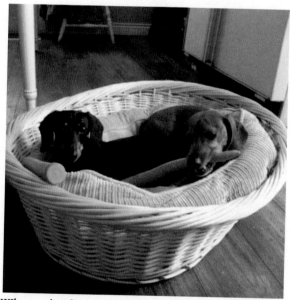

Who needs a bone to clean teeth when you have carrots!

Chapter 5: Gerson Cookbook
aka Survival Guide

"Let food be thy medicine and medicine be thy food."
Hippocrates

So You Think You <u>CAN'T</u> Cook...

Do not think you have to be a good cook to enjoy scrumptious meals while doing the Gerson Therapy.

I've come to realize that I am not good at cooking... at all! Just ask my family and friends. In fact, I have used the oven more since being on the Gerson Therapy than I have my entire life! My talent is in combining ingredients (maybe taking good photos helps too).

Sometimes all it takes to ignite the creative cook inside of us is to browse over some inspiring photographs. So I have included many pictures because you might find that you don't even need a recipe once you get ideas of how to put together Gerson - friendly ingredients. And if you need a step by step recipe, they are there too.

Enjoy.

RECIPE INDEX

Gerson Therapy Approved Herbs

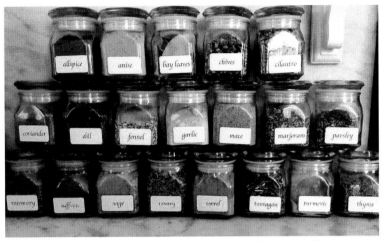

...photograph by Stacie Coburn

Extract from "Healing the Gerson Way" by Charlotte Gerson, daughter of Dr Max Gerson (available from the Gerson Institute www.gerson.org and also on Amazon).

Many spices are high in aromatic acids, which are irritants and are likely to counteract the healing reaction. This is why only the following mild spices are permitted, to be used in very small doses:

- allspice
- anise
- bay leaves
- coriander
- dill
- fennel
- mace
- marjoram
- rosemary

- saffron
- sage
- sorrel
- summer savory
- tarragon
- thyme
- And ... Turmeric. Though not yet 'approved', but based on the strong evidence of its benefits the Gerson Institute says you can use turmeric.

NOTE: chives, garlic, onion and parsley may be used in larger amounts.

Substitutions

If your favorite herb is not on the allowable list, this might help...

- allspice is a good substitute for cinnamon, cloves or nutmeg
- Mace is similar to nutmeg
- Saffron can substitute for turmeric especially for color
- Marjoram could replace Basil
- Thyme instead of basil and oregano

BREAKFAST

Truffle Porridge

This is my breakfast. It's like eating truffle, digging into the custard to expose the fruit sweetened creamy oats.

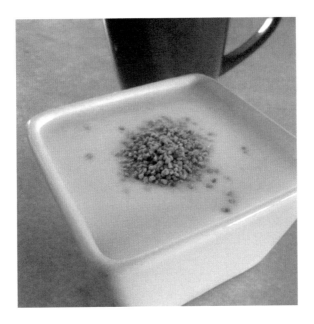

You'll need;
1/4 cup whole organic oats

1/2 cup water

Spoonful of dried unsulphured organic fruit

Gerson Custard (see recipe)

Sprinkling of bee pollen (optional)

NOTE: Bee pollen can only added after several weeks on Gerson Therapy and when recommended by your practitioner.

Method

1. Pre-soak oats in water overnight with some organic dried fruit.
2. Slow cook it, still in the dish, in a slow cooker. Or over low heat in a saucepan.
3. Leave to cool to eating temperature before topping with Gerson 'custard' and bee pollen.

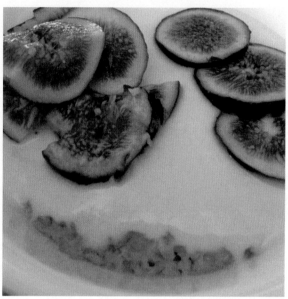

Give your oats variety by adding different organic fruits like these figs.

Easy Pancakes

Recipe by *Jeanette Nazario*

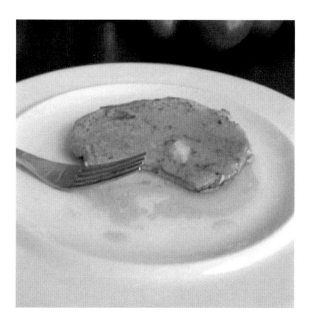

You'll need;

1/2 cup oatmeal (ground to flour consistency in a blender or mill)
1/2 green apple made into sauce
Distilled water

Method

1. Mix together oatmeal and apple with water until it reaches pancake batter consistency.
2. Before dropping into pan, sprinkle a few drops of distilled water and put the mix in, before the water evaporates.
3. You might need to keep adding a few drops of water here and there, so it won't stick.
4. Drizzle with organic maple syrup and a dollop of drained non-fat yogurt (if allowed).

Oatmeal Pancakes

Recipe by *Beth Perera*

For this recipe you make oat milk by straining the oats through a fine mesh stainless strainer which might be useful for if you need a milk replacement.

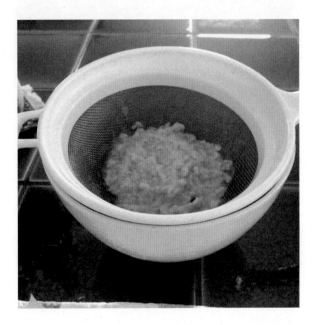

You'll need:

5 cups pure water
2 1/2 cups oats
Applesauce
Maple syrup

Method

1. Soak the 1/2 a cup of oats in the water for 10 minutes.
2. Blend on high for 1 minute.
3. Strain the oats through a fine mesh stainless strainer (or cheesecloth). Store oat milk in glass container (keeps well for 3-4

days). You will need 1 ½ cups of the oat milk for the pancake batter.

4. To make oat "flour," put remaining 2 cups of oats in Vitamix and blend on setting 4 until finely processed. (You can also use a blender or food processor)

5. Combine oat flour with 1 ½ cups oat milk and your applesauce.

6. Drop onto hot griddle. Flip pancakes when top side appears bubbly and edges are visibly cooked (a couple minutes on each side usually does the trick).

Note: To heat the maple syrup, place glass container of syrup in a slightly larger bowl of hot water.

Pikelets

This is a nice alternative for breakfast. They will not rise but kind of 'set'. Serve hot or cold with strained non-fat yogurt (if allowed).

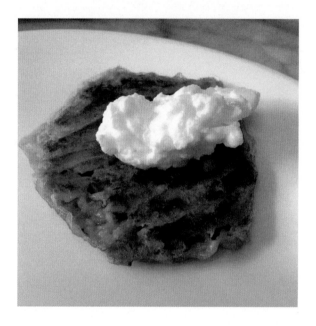

You'll need:

2/3 cup well strained cooked oats

1 small mashed banana

1 tablespoon cranberries (or other dried fruit)

1 tablespoon raw oats or oat flour

Method

1. Mix all together adding extra raw oats or flour if mixture too runny.
2. Place teaspoons of mixture on baking paper and cook at 350°F (180°C) for 25 minutes. They might not look cooked.
3. Once cooked peel off paper gently to reveal browned side and turn over to cool a bit to firm up.

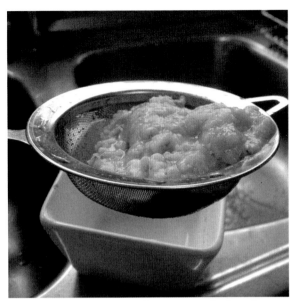

Straining excess water from oats to thicken them.

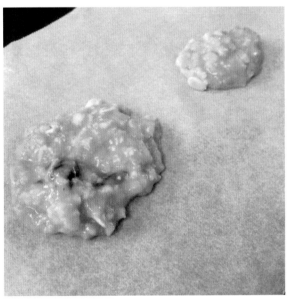

Place teaspoons of mixture on baking paper.

COOL MEALS

Cilantro Summer Potato

If you're wanting something fresh, tasty (kinda salty) and crunchy, you'll love this. It is also great if your baked potato is too hot to eat and needs cooling down.

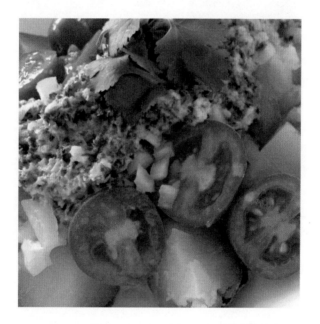

You'll need:
1 large baked potato
2 stalks celery finely chopped
8 cherry tomatoes (or 2 regular)
Chopped bunch of fresh cilantro
1/3 cup non-fat yogurt
1 teaspoon flaxseed oil

Method

1. Bake potato for 1 hour at 350°F (180°C).
2. Blender add cilantro, non-fat yogurt and oil in a blender.
3. Cut open baked potato and put in big bowl. Top with raw tomato and celery.
4. Pour over cilantro dressing.

NOTE: The cilantro mush settles on top while a non-fat yogurt sauce drizzles to bottom, almost like a soup.

IMPORTANT: A non-fat yogurt allowance is only added after several weeks on Gerson Therapy and when recommended by your practitioner.

Crunchy Tangy Potato Salad

Warning: Don't mix this up to serve it! Looks disgusting mixed up. But tastes amazing!

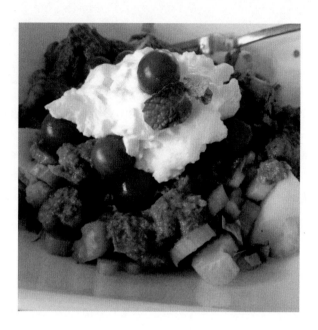

You'll need;
Cold potatoes chopped

Mint chopped

Celery sliced

Grapefruit and cilantro dressing (or your favorite)

Cherry tomatoes (whole)

Drained non-fat yogurt (generous scoop)

Garnish (very important!) of tomato and sprig of mint

Method

1. Place ingredients into a dish in the order listed.

IMPORTANT: A non-fat yogurt allowance is only added after several weeks on Gerson Therapy and when recommended by your practitioner.

Jfur's Gerson Slaw

Recipe by *Jennifer Simpson*

This is one of my goto dishes. Great to use by itself or as an addition to many other dishes. Makes a great addition to green salad, great topping for a baked potato, as part of a veggie wrap or quinoa dish. I even like to mix it in my mashed potatoes or rosemary-honey potato wedges. In fact, add cubed cooked potatoes and you have a ready potato salad. Experiment with the flavors and the veggies that you like best. I try to keep a batch in my fridge so I have a ready, raw veggie addition to any meal, and I like that it uses produce I always have on hand anyway!

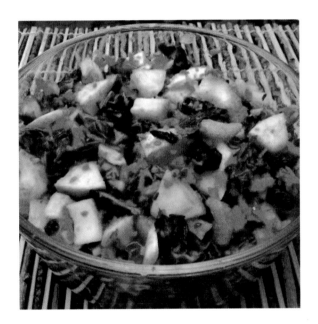

You'll need;
2-3 inch slice of red cabbage

1/2 med onion

1/4-1/2 cup raisins (sulphur free and organic)

1 apple (I like green)

2 med carrots

2 celery stalks

Apple cider vinegar to taste (approx ½ cup?)

Method

1. Combine raisins and apple cider vinegar into a large bowl. Let the raisins sit in the vinegar while you make the 'slaw' to help reconstitute them (dried fruit needs to be reconstituted on the Gerson Therapy). The juices from the other produce will also help as the 'slaw' sits in fridge.

    FOR NORWALK USERS:
2. Cut cabbage, carrots and onion to fit in shoot.
3. Place bowl under shoot.
4. Using NO grid, fill shoot with cabbage pieces and place pusher in shoot.
5. Turn on machine and push cabbage through as quickly as possible (for best results).
6. Turn off machine.
7. Do the same process with the onions.
8. Then place largest grid (#0) in grid holder.
9. Load carrots in shoot. (Remember to place pusher in shoot before turning on machine). Push carrots through shoot as quickly as possible. (Too slow makes them too pulpy and not like diced carrots).

    NOTE: All of the above can be done using a food processor or hand grater. These are just tricks I have learned using the Norwalk, which I find easier to use and clean (if you've got it, might as well use it). However, I prefer to prepare the apple and celery by hand as the Norwalk doesn't do a good job with these.

10. Slice, core, and cut apple into small pieces (an apple corer/slicer helps the Gerson Person tremendously).
11. Cut celery into small pieces.

12. Mix all ingredients together and place in bowl with lid (I use a 2 quart/litre Pyrex bowl).
13. Let sit in fridge for several hours.

    Enjoy!

Lettuce Wrap

Serve with a serve of Gerson Wedges and your friends will be saying... "I'll have what she's having!"

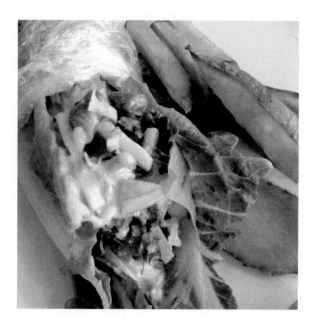

You'll need;
Two large cos lettuce leaves
Drained low-fat yogurt (optional if allowed)
Your favorite salad
Your favorite dressing
Cling wrap (Yes I know it's plastic but it's not on there for long. Just doesn't work well with baking paper.)

Method

1. First place a large sheet of wrap over a plate. Put the lettuce leaves on wrap side by side making sure some sticks out on top (where

you'll bite into it) and that there is plenty of excess at the bottom.

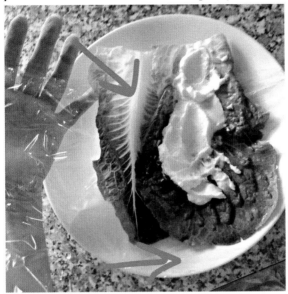

2. Spread with yogurt (optional) then salad and dressing.
3. Fold over the wrap from the side first, rolling up lettuce as you go. Then with other hand fold up bottom (this will catch all the yummy juices). Finally fold over other side.

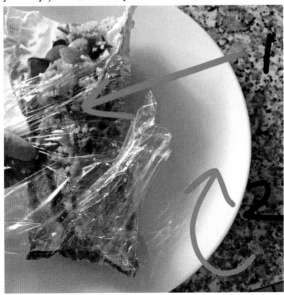

4. Serve with potatoes and soup. Make sure you have a napkin handy. A pile of them!

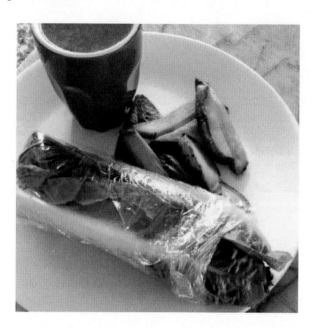

Subway Gerson Therapy Style

This is just like eating a crusty roll. Enjoy hot or cold.

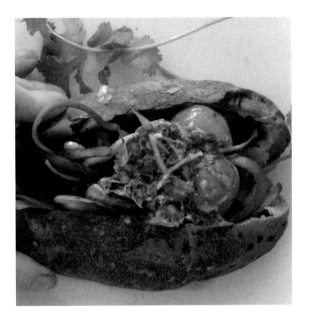

You'll need;
Large potato (roll shaped)
Your favorite mix of salad
Your favorite dressing

Method

1. Bake potato for 1 hour at 200°F (100°C). Or until knife goes in easily. If you like it really crispy, try baking for an extra 30 minutes at 350°F (180°C). Of course ovens vary. Let cool.
2. Cut in half trying to leave hinged at bottom. Scoop out cooked potato which you can eat separately.
3. Fill with salad and top with dressing.

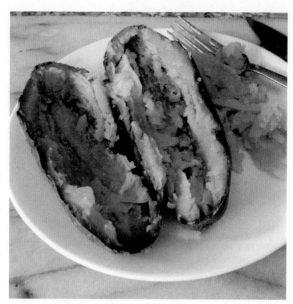

A scooped out cold baked potato is your crusty roll.

Sweet'n'Tangy Tato

First, let me introduce you to sorrel. If you've already met, you'll know how surprising this herb tastes. It is a herb that you can also use as a lettuce. It has a lemony tangy taste. The first time I tasted it, I thought I had had lemon juice on my fingers that got onto the sorrel.

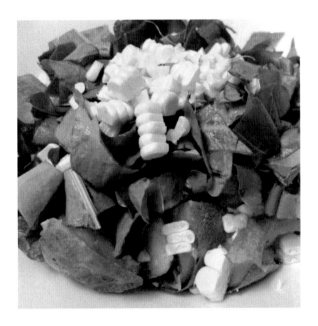

You'll need:
1 baked potato
1 bunch of sorrel (or cos lettuce)
1 corn cob
Gerson Therapy dressing (see recipe)

Method

1. Cut open potato and top with chopped sorrel and raw corn kernels.
2. Pour over dressing.

HOT MEALS

Frittata Gerson Therapy Style

No eggs of course! This is an easy 'chuck it all together' country style meal. Good one for entertaining with friends. Even your non - Gerson friends will drool over it. You will NEED a food processor or a slicer thingo though.

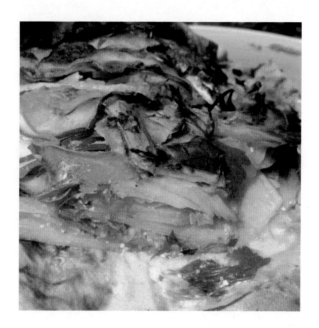

You'll need:

4 potatoes

3 tomatoes

1 zucchini

1/2 onion

Fresh parsley

1/4 cup non-fat yogurt

Method

1. In a food processor slice all veggies. Roughly chop parsley.
2. Mix in non-fat yogurt.
3. Line a loaf pan generously with baking paper. Spoon in veggies.
4. Bake for 45 minutes in oven set to 300°F (150°C) or until cooked (knife goes through easily) and brown on top.
5. Pull out of tin by paper and serve while still in paper on a board or large plate.

IMPORTANT: A non-fat yogurt allowance is only added after several weeks on Gerson Therapy and when recommended by your practitioner.

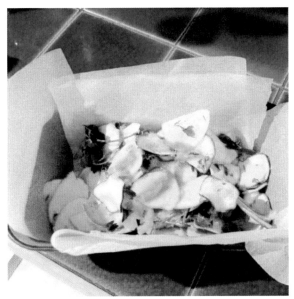

Line a loaf pan generously with baking paper.

Gerson Therapy Parfait

You can't SEE how yummy this was (next time I'll put it in a glass jar) but trust me, it was!

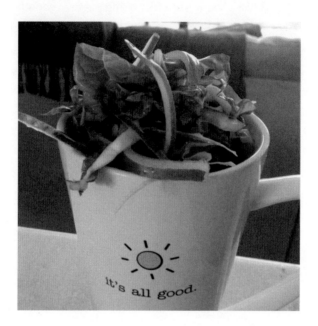

You'll need:

1 baked potato

1 handful of shredded crisp cabbage or lettuce

1 tomato chopped

1 stalk celery finely chopped (or red onion)

Non-fat yogurt

Flaxseed oil/lemon/honey dressing

Method

1. Smash hot potatoes and put in tall mug.
2. Add non-fat yogurt to cover.
3. Add half chopped tomato.
4. Add celery/onion.

5. Add lettuce and rest of tomato.

6. Pour dressing over and … eat enjoying the different tastes, textures and temperatures.

IMPORTANT: A non-fat yogurt allowance is only added after several weeks on Gerson Therapy and when recommended by your practitioner.

Beet Pasta

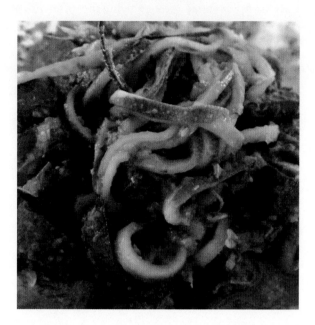

You'll need:

2 tomatoes

Rosemary or other Gerson approved fresh herb

1 beetroot

1 potato

Bunch parsley

2 celery sticks

Garlic to taste

2 teaspoons flaxseed oil

Method

1. Chop tomatoes and put in oven-proof dish, sprinkle with herbs. Cube potatoes and beets. Place on baking paper. Bake for 30 minutes at 350°F (180°C).
2. Use spiraller on zucchinis or grate. (If you'd like warm 'pasta' place in oven)

3. Sauce: Into blender add cooked tomatoes, parsley, garlic, flaxseed oil and celery. Blend.
4. Gently mix zucchini pasta with roasted beets, potatoes and sauce.

Beetroot Delish

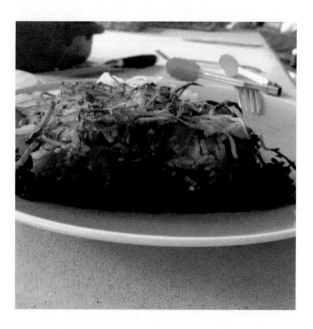

You'll need:

4 beetroots

1 cup cherry tomatoes

2 potatoes

1 orange

Bunch fresh mint

Rosemary or other Gerson approved herb

1 teaspoon honey

Method

1. Grate unpeeled potatoes in food processor. Mix in rosemary and put aside. (Do this before beets because it will be beet red after)
2. Grate beets in food processor. (Peel if your beets are bitter)
3. Quarter orange and process in a food processor.
4. Add chopped mint and honey to beet mixture.

5. Line loaf tin with double layer of baking paper and spoon in beet mix.
6. Place whole tomatoes in a layer on top. Pierce each with a knife to prevent exploding.
7. Top with grated potato mix and bake at 350°F (180°C) for 30 minutes.

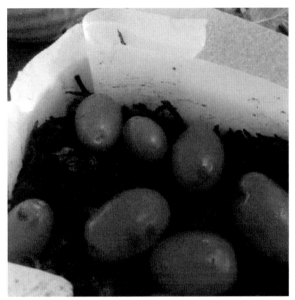

Place whole tomatoes in a layer. Pierce each with a knife to prevent exploding.

Warning: Beet juice stains. Be extra careful as it gets messy. And the colorful CE next day is a bonus!

Creamy Cauliflower Soup

Recipe by *Jfur Simpson*

This is a great one to serve if you are eating with a non-Gerson Therapy person and they'll never know.

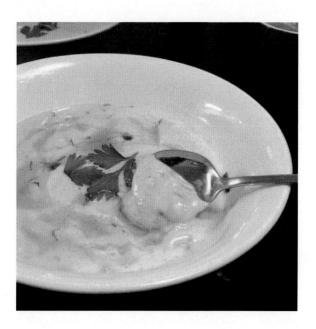

You'll need:

Half a cauliflower

2 medium unpeeled potatoes

Parsley - chopped (a lot or a little depending on your taste buds)

2 tablespoons flaxseed oil

1 tablespoon apple cider vinegar (optional)

Raw honey to drizzle (optional)

Method

1. Slow cook potatoes and cauliflower until soft. (Might be a bit smelly)

2. Place cooled veggies in a blender cover with cool water, add vinegar. Blend on high until smooth.
3. Now the technique that makes it SO creamy. Blend on low/med speed and carefully take lid off while still running (or if you're lucky there's a hole in the lid) and slowly pour in flaxseed oil. You will see the consistency change from mashed veggie texture to smooth and creamy. **IMPORTANT:** Soup must not be too hot when you add flaxseed oil or you will destroy its qualities. That's why you add cool water to blend.
4. Put the parsley in serving bowls (heat them if you like) and pour soup in. Garnish with a parsley sprig and drizzle honey on the surface. Enjoy!

TIP: Cook the veggies in advance and let them go cold. When you blend add boiling water.

Variations

- Blend parsley with cauliflower for a 'green' soup.
- Try other veggies like broccoli but doesn't seem to get quite as creamy.
- Add 1/2 yellow onion, 1 clove garlic, and some chopped celery (for sodium) to the pot with the potatoes and cauliflower.
- Try adding a touch of fennel powder once it is puréed.

Mash As A Meal

Yes there is comfort food on Gerson. Imagine cuddled up on the couch watching a movie with a big warm bowl of this!

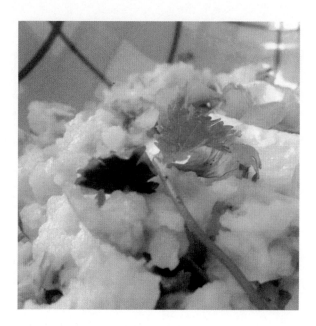

You'll need;
3 medium potatoes
2 stalks celery
Bunch of cilantro (you'll only use the stems)
1/2 cup non fat yogurt
1 tablespoon flaxseed oil

Method

1. Wash and chop potatoes. Boil with skin on.
2. Finely dice celery and cilantro stems (these provide crunch).
3. Drain potatoes and mash well with yogurt.
4. Mix in flaxseed oil thoroughly (potatoes are cooled by yogurt so heat will not destroy flaxseed properties).

5. Stir in celery and cilantro. Serve with an extra dollop of yogurt!

IMPORTANT: A non-fat yogurt allowance is only added after several weeks on Gerson Therapy and when recommended by your practitioner.

Easy Winter Casserole

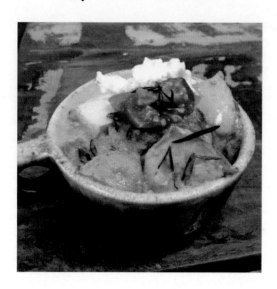

You'll need;

Potatoes

Tomatoes

Onion

Rosemary (fresh if available)

Non-fat yogurt

Method

1. Put roughly chopped unpeeled potatoes on baking paper into moderate oven.
2. Put halved tomatoes, chopped onion and rosemary in a covered oven-proof dish and into oven with potatoes.
3. Cook until potatoes cooked.
4. Mix together with non-fat yogurt and serve.
5. Top with a dollop of drained non-fat yogurt to serve.

IMPORTANT: A non-fat yogurt allowance is only added after several weeks on Gerson Therapy and when recommended by your practitioner.

Hippocrates Soup

This is Dr Max Gerson's original special soup recipe, named after the father of modern medicine.

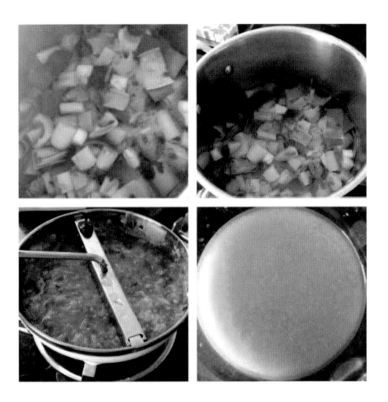

You'll need;
1 medium celery knob (or 3-4 stalks of celery stalks)

1 medium parsley root (rarely available; may be omitted)

2 small leeks or one large leek (if not available, use 2 small onions instead)

2 medium onions

Garlic as desired (may also be squeezed raw into the hot soup instead of cooking it)

Small amount of parsley

750g (1-1/2 pounds) tomatoes (approx 6 or more, if desired)

500g (1 pound potatoes) (approx 4)

Method

1. Wash and scrub vegetables and cut into slices or 1/2-inch cubes.
2. Put in large pot, add water to just cover vegetables, bring to a boil, then cook slowly on low heat for 1-1/2 to 2 hours until all the vegetables are soft.
3. Pass through a food mill to remove fibers. Let soup cool before storing in refrigerator.

IMPORTANT: Do not add or substitute ingredients.

Hippocrates Stew

Most importantly serve this meal on nice china, and eat with someone you love!

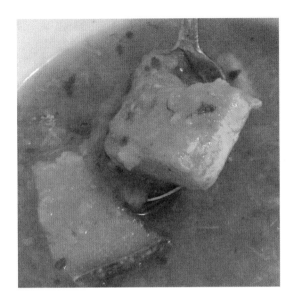

You'll need;
Cauliflower
Broccoli
Zucchini
Pumpkin
Honey/Apple cider vinegar/flaxseed oil dressing (optional)

Method

1. Place cauliflower, zucchini and broccoli in a slow cooker (approx 2 hours).
2. Cut pumpkin into 1/3 inch slices (keep peel on). Place on a try lined with baking paper.
3. Bake at 350°F (180°C) for 45 minutes.
4. Pour over a cup of Hippocrates soup.
5. Pour over the dressing once on the plate.

Smashed Easy Veg

Smashing veggies is really just a modern way of lazy mashing! A country chunky texture is the result.

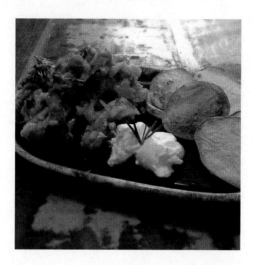

You'll need;
Cauliflower
Pumpkin (Jap if available)
One tomato
Potatoes

Method

1. Place cauliflower pieces, sliced pumpkin (with peel on), thickly sliced potatoes and the tomato (whole) on baking paper.
2. Cook for 1 hour 15 minutes on 350°F (180°C).
3. 'Smash' cauliflower, pumpkin and tomato together. Be careful as the tomato juices are hot and can splatter.
4. Serve with drained non-fat yogurt.

IMPORTANT: A non-fat yogurt allowance is only added after several weeks on Gerson Therapy and when recommended by your practitioner.

Spaghetti Carbonara Gerson Style

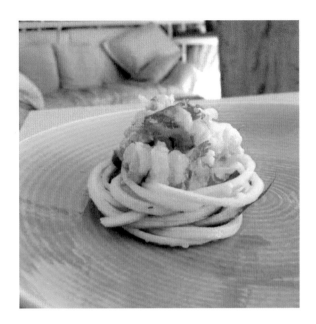

You'll need:

2 medium potatoes

1 bunch cilantro

6 stalks celery

1 zucchini

½ cup non-fat yogurt

2 teaspoon flaxseed oil

½ onion (optional)

Garlic to taste (optional)

Method

1. Boil unpeeled, chopped potatoes until soft.
2. Chop celery, onion, garlic and cilantro finely. Using vegetable spiraller turn zucchini into spaghetti (or grate/chop and place in serving bowls.

3. Drain potatoes and roughly mash (leave chunky style). Add non-fat yogurt until blended.
4. Stir in flaxseed oil, cilantro, celery etc.
5. Spoon on top of zucchini spaghetti and serve.

IMPORTANT: A non-fat yogurt allowance is only added after several weeks on Gerson Therapy and when recommended by your practitioner.

Veg-hetti Bolognaise

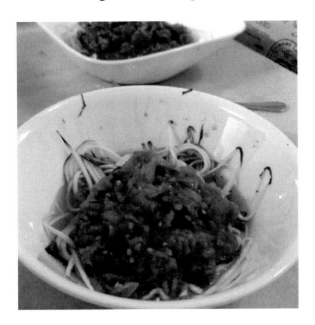

You'll need:
1 onion
5 tomatoes
1 bunch parsley
Garlic to taste
3 zucchinis

Method

1. Roughly chop onion, tomatoes and parsley and slow cook with garlic until tender. About 1 ½ hours.
2. Turn zucchini into spaghetti and place in oven to warm. Do not cover or it will become mush.
3. When sauce is cooked mash with a potato masher (not blender) for a chunky texture sauce.

Gersghetti

The smell of this is just as good (I think better) than an authentic Italian pasta cooking. The addition of potatoes makes this a complete Gerson meal that the whole family will enjoy. My 10 year old puts this in his top five favorite meals!

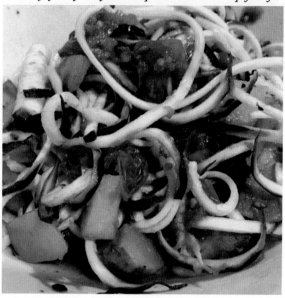

You'll need:
6 medium tomatoes

4 medium potatoes

2 sticks celery

Sprig fresh thyme (1/4 teaspoon if dried)

Garlic to taste, chopped

3 zucchini

1 tablespoon flaxseed oil

Method

1. Finely chop unpeeled potatoes and celery. Quarter tomatoes. Add to oven proof dish with thyme, garlic and one tablespoon water.

2. Cook covered at 260°F (130°C) for 120 minutes. Stirring half way through.
3. Spiralize zucchini (no gadget? then grate or use vegetable peeler).
4. Remove from oven and mix raw zucchini immediately.
5. Tosh through flaxseed oil before serving.

Gerson Baked Spaghetti

Recipe by an "awesome" Gerson person

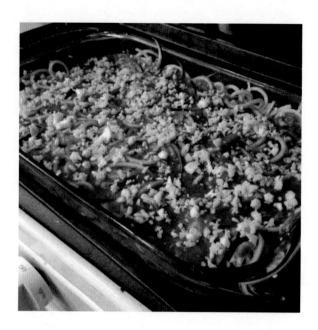

You'll need;
3 medium zucchini
2 tomatoes
1 medium-large onion
Several cloves of garlic
¼ cup grated cauliflower
Handful of parsley

Method

1. Roast tomatoes, onions, and garlic in the oven until tomatoes release juices and everything is very soft. Remove and blend into sauce.
2. Add parsley or other desired/allowed herbs.

3. While veggies are roasting, spiralize zucchini into "noodles" and place into baking dish.
4. Pulse cauliflower in food processor to grate it and make it look like shredded cheese.
5. Top "Zoodles" with sauce and grated cauliflower. Place back into oven until tender, or eat raw.

Variation: Slice the zucchini into wide strips for layering. Using the same sauce and sliced or crumbled cauliflower, create layers as if you were making lasagne. Bake and you've got a lasagne.

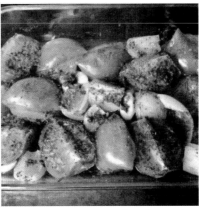

Roast tomatoes, onions, and garlic in the oven.

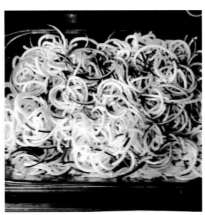

Zucchini turned into "Zoodles".

Quinoa al Pomodoro di Maria

Recipe by *Doris Parreno*

So what does "Quinoa al Pomodoro di Maria" mean? It's Italian for "Maria's quinoa in a tomato sauce!" In Italian it just sounds more romantic!

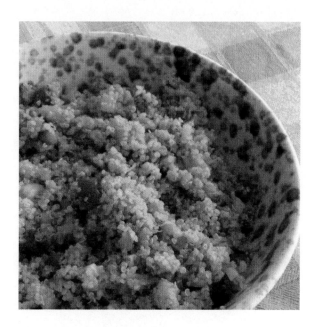

You'll need;
1 onion finely chopped
2 cloves garlic finely chopped
2 tomatoes finely chopped
2 cups washed organic quinoa
3 cups distilled water
1 tablespoon flaxseed oil
Parsley to taste

Method

1. Sauté in water onion, garlic, tomatoes and parsley over low heat until golden.

2. Add quinoa and sauté for 1 minute.
3. Add 3 cups of water and let simmer in low. When water evaporates it is done.
4. Once cooked and cooled slightly, drizzle with flaxseed oil (flaxseed oil never to be added to hot food as its qualities are heat sensitive. Adding to warm food is ok.).

Veggo Pizza

You'll need a food processor or slicing gadget for this. It's yummy but don't convince your kids it's traditional pizza. Call it veggie pie if you make it for Pizza Hut lovers.

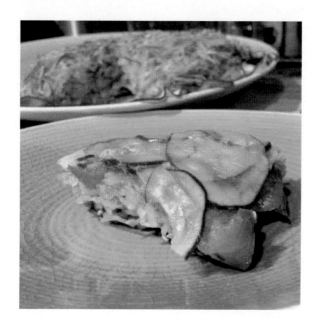

You'll need:
1 large zucchini
3 medium tomatoes
Bunch fresh parsley
Garlic
2 medium potatoes

Method

1. Slice zucchini thinly.
2. Place a double layer of baking paper on a cooling rack on an oven tray (so heat can get under).
3. Arrange zucchini in a circle. This is pizza base.

4. Slice tomatoes. Mix in finely chopped parsley and garlic. This is pizza sauce. Spread over zucchini base leaving about an inch of the zucchini base uncovered at the edges.

5. Finely grate potatoes and pile on top. This is the cheese so pile it up!

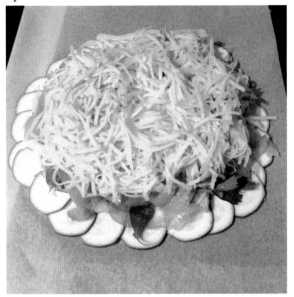

6. Cook for 30 minutes at 350°F (180°C).

TIP: To remove baking paper place a plate on top of pizza and turn over quickly. Gently peel off paper. Then using another plate flip to the right side up. And… seems it is easier to eat upside down, potato side down!

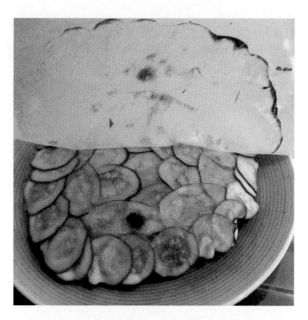

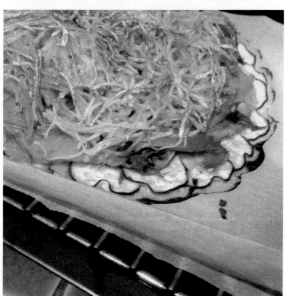

Cook on a double layer of baking paper on a cooling rack so heat can get under.

Stuffed Zucchini

Recipe by *Shelley Food Angel*

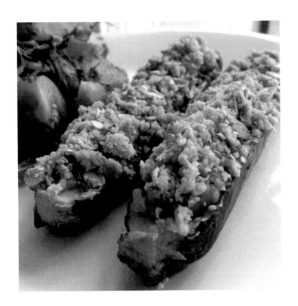

You'll need:

2 small evenly sized zucchinis

1 cup pumpkin or large potato

1 onion

Oats

Garlic to taste

Method

1. Cook zucchini and pumpkin (or potato).
2. Cut zucchini in half and scoop out inside.
3. Cook onion, garlic and zucchini insides. Add cooked pumpkin or potato and mash with onion mixture.
4. Stuff shelled out zucchinis with mashed mixture. Top with blended oats.
5. Bake in oven at 350°F (180°C) until browned.

Tomato Parsley Spaghetti with
Honey Rosemary Potatoes

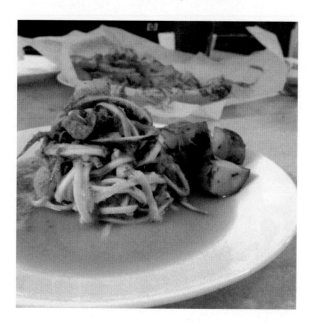

You'll need:

2 whole tomatoes

Bunch of fresh parsley

2 celery stalks

1 medium zucchini

Garlic to taste

3 potatoes

Rosemary (fresh preferably)

2 teaspoons raw honey

Method

1. Place whole tomatoes into oven proof dish into a 350°F (180°C) oven. Put timer on for 30 minutes.

2. Cut unpeeled potatoes into chunks. Finely chop rosemary.

3. Mix together with honey (dissolve honey first into some hot water if cold weather solidifies it) to cover potatoes and tip onto a baking paper covered tray. Put in oven with tomatoes.

4. Use a spiraller to turn zucchini into spaghetti (or grate). Put into oven proof dish and into oven. Do not cover or zucchini will lose spaghetti shape and go to mash.

5. When tomatoes are cooked remove from oven and reset timer for another 30 minutes or until potatoes are cooked.

6. Put cooked tomatoes into a blender with parsley, roughly chopped celery and garlic, blending until smooth.

7. Take warmed zucchini from oven and mix sauce through. Serve with potatoes.

Zucchini Noodle Casserole

Recipe by *Betsy Gahn*

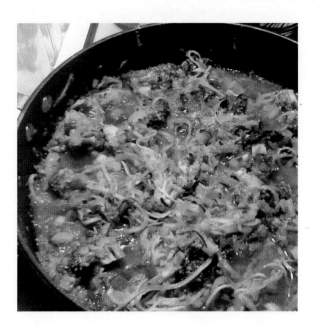

You'll need:
3 zucchinis
Bunch broccoli
1 green onion or shallot
1 yellow bell pepper
Fresh dill
Garlic
Sauce:
2 tomatoes
2 green onions
Small sweet orange pepper

Method

1. Sautée dill and garlic in a bit of water in large pan.

2. Put zucchini spaghetti in pan.
3. Add onion, broccoli and pepper in pan and simmer slowly.
4. Sauce: cook sauce ingredients in small saucepan until water cooks off.
5. Add sauce to cooked vegetables and serve.

Cauliflower Baked

One night I couldn't be bothered cutting the cauliflower up (one of 'those' days) so put it in the oven whole! Looked great and tasted fab and there's a soft delicious centre with crunchy brown ends!

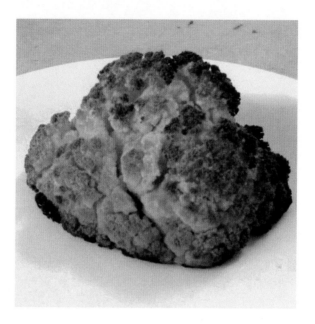

You'll need:

Half a cauliflower

Method

1. Put cauliflower on baking/parchment paper on oven tray.
2. Bake at 350°F (180°C) for about an hour until golden.

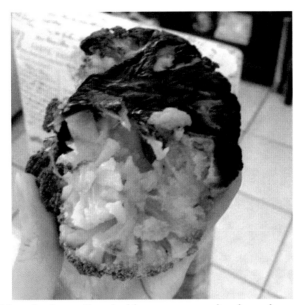

Note that's a well cooked bottom, caramelized, not burned.

Creamy Crunchy Cheesey Potatoes

This is just like eating cream cheese! Seriously. Of course it's not.

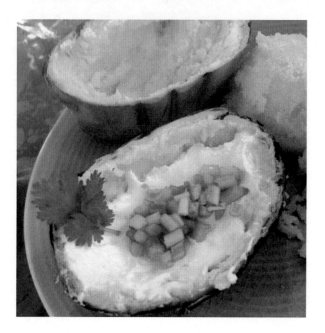

You'll need:

Non-fat yogurt

Onion finely chopped

Cilantro stems

Baked potatoes

Method

1. Strain non-fat yogurt overnight through a cheese cloth (or tea/dish towel).
2. Discard the whey.
3. Mix with finely chopped onion and/or chopped cilantro stems as they have the most flavor and crunch too!

4. Scoop out halved baked potatoes and fill with non-fat yogurt mixture.
5. Top with extra cilantro.

IMPORTANT: A non-fat yogurt allowance is only added after several weeks on Gerson Therapy and when recommended by your practitioner.

Potatoes and Spinach

Recipe by *Doris Parreno*

This is a great cook and serve in the same dish.

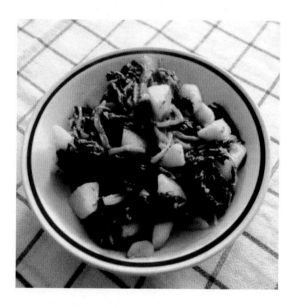

You'll need;

3 potatoes

½ onion

3 cloves garlic

3 cups spinach

1 cup water

1 tablespoon flaxseed oil

Method

1. Sauté onion and garlic in a bit of water for 2 minutes.
2. Add chopped spinach and 1 cup of water, cover with lid and cook on low for 20 minutes.
3. Let cool slightly and serve with sprinkle of flaxseed oil on top. If allowed, try adding a big dollop of drained non-fat yogurt too.

Beetroot Fries

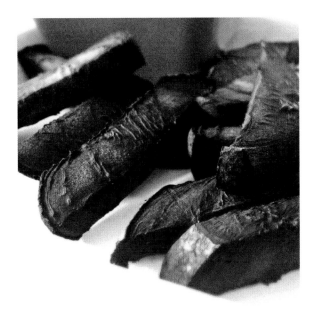

You'll need:

Beetroot

Method

1. Wash but do not peel. Cut into chunky strips and place on baking paper.
2. Bake in oven at 300°F (150°C) for 45 minutes or until cooked.

TIP: If you want them a bit crisper, pop under the grill for 5 minutes to finish but realize this may destroy nutrients.

Herbed Potatoes

These are my family movie night snack. Place them in front of the kids and I bet they'll eat them too.

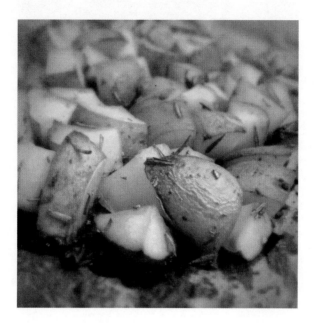

You'll need:
Potatoes, unpeeled and sliced
Your favorite Gerson Therapy approved herbs (Rosemary used in photo)

Method

1. Place potatoes on baking paper.
2. Sprinkle with herbs while still wet.
3. Bake in oven 300°F (150°C) for 45 minutes.

TIP: If you want them a bit browner, pop under the grill for 5 minutes to finish.

Potato Herb Crunch

Super easy recipe when you're needing a different way of eating potatoes. Also a nice one to share with friends dipped into drained non-fat yogurt (if allowed).

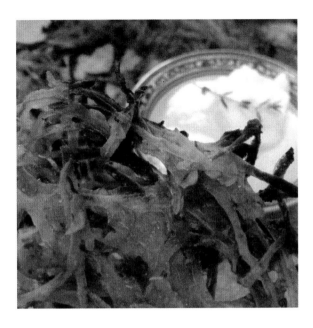

You'll need:
4 washed unpeeled potatoes
Fresh rosemary and thyme (or your favorite herbs)
2 teaspoons honey

Method

1. Grate potatoes and finely chop herbs. A food processor is handy.
2. Mix together and place on baking paper gently. Do not flatten.
3. Bake 30 minutes at 425°F (220°C) until brown and cooked.

TIP: Try adding fennel seeds for bursts of flavor.

Potato Patties

Recipe by *Shelly Food Angel*

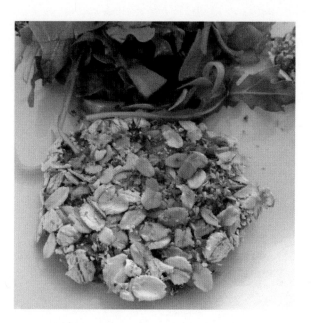

You'll need:

1 Sebago potato

1 carrot cut into thin strips

1 zucchini cut into thin strips

1 onion diced

1 clove of garlic diced

Oats

Dried thyme

Method

1. Steam the potato until just soft.
2. Blend the potato. Then add the cut vegetables, onion and garlic.
3. Blend some oats with a little dried thyme.
4. Sprinkle oat flour onto a baking tray so the patties won't stick.

5. Mix together with the potato mix and make small patties and place on a baking tray.
6. Sprinkle oat flour on top of patties.
7. Bake until crispy and browned on top.

Gerson Wedges

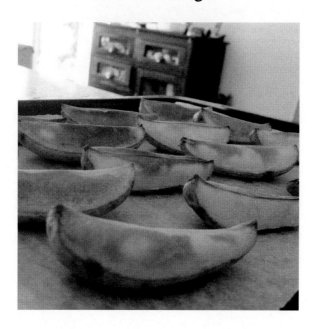

You'll need;

Potatoes

Method

1. Cut washed but not peeled potatoes into wedged shaped fries.
2. Spread on baking paper on baking tray.
3. Cook in oven at 350°F (180°C) for about 45 minutes until brown
4. Serve in a cup and (if allowed) with "sour cream" (aka drained low-fat yogurt) on the side.

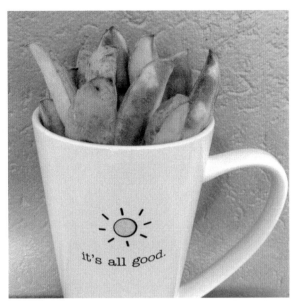

NOTE: this way of baking (in small pieces) is allowed on holidays or special occasions only since it exposes too much potato surface to the heat, destroying too many nutrients in potatoes. The whole baked potato is still the best way to get the nutrients so remains a regular at meal times.

Gerson Rosti 'Pull-A-Part'

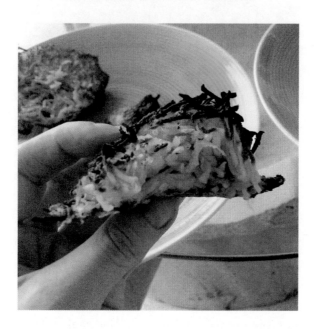

You'll need:

3 medium potatoes washed

½ onion

2 sprigs fresh rosemary (or your favorite Gerson-approved herbs)

1 tablespoon non-fat yogurt

2 teaspoons honey

Method

1. Grate potatoes and onion on fine setting (I use a food processor).
2. Chop herbs and mix with honey and non-fat yogurt (or chuck it all into a bullet blender).
3. For a 'pull-a-part' style to share, pile evenly on to baking paper in a rough loaf shape about an inch high. For a 'crisp on the outside, soft on the inside' individual serve, place into rough balls.

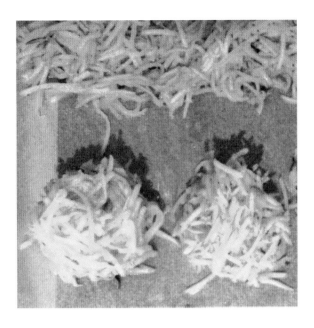

4. Bake for 30 minutes at 350°F (180°C) or until brown. Leave
    longer if you like crispy!

NOTE: this way of baking (in small pieces) is allowed on holidays or
special occasions only since it exposes too much potato surface to the heat,
destroying too many nutrients in potatoes. The whole baked potato is still
the best way to get the nutrients so remains a regular at meal times.

IMPORTANT: A non-fat yogurt allowance is only added after several
weeks on Gerson Therapy and when recommended by your practitioner.

Roasted Cauliflower Rice

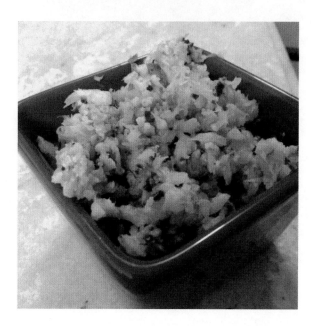

You'll need;
Cauliflower

Method

1. Cut cauliflower into small pieces.
2. Spread on baking paper on baking tray.
3. Cook in oven at 350°F (180°C) for about an hour. The cauliflower will brown beautifully in the oven.
4. Mash lightly with a potato masher until it looks like rice.

Roasted Pumpkin Potato

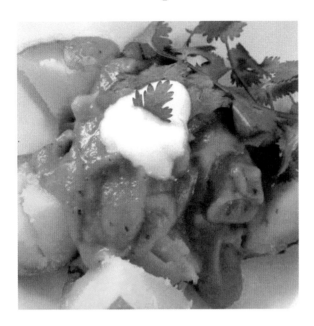

You'll need:

Large potato

Pumpkin cut into thin wedges leaving peel on

Method

1. Bake potato (about 1 hour at 350°F (180°C)).
2. Roast pumpkin on baking paper (About 45 minutes at 350°F (180°C)).
3. Blend or mash cooked pumpkin with enough hot water until smooth.
4. Pour over smashed potato, topping with non-fat yogurt (if allowed) and cilantro.

Cauliflower and Celery Salad

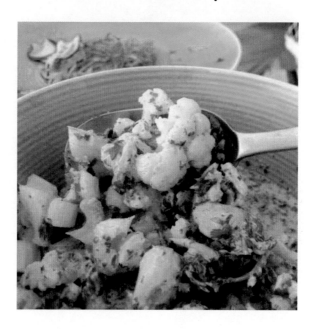

You'll need;
Cauliflower
Celery
Dressing:
Non-fat yogurt
Flaxseed oil
Bunch cilantro

Method

1. Cut cauliflower into small pieces and cook. Leave to cool.
2. Add finely chopped celery.
3. Bend together dressing ingredients and mix in.

IMPORTANT: A non-fat yogurt allowance is only added after several weeks on Gerson Therapy and when recommended by your practitioner.

DRESSING AND SAUCES

Cauliflower Sauce

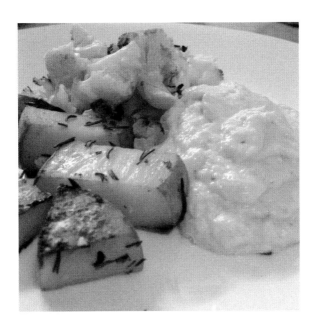

You'll need;
A serving of Creamy Cauliflower Soup

Method

1. Ah ha! A soup now becomes a sauce. Serve it over potatoes or any vegetables.

Celery Cilantro Lime Dressing

This one is a goodie to disguise the taste of flaxseed oil and bee pollen. Use it over a salad or even a cooked dish to cool it down.

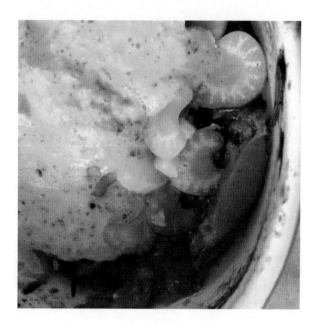

You'll need;

Fresh cilantro

Half a lime (lemon if you like it really tangy), peel and seeds removed

2 sticks of celery, roughly chopped

1 tablespoon flaxseed oil

1 tablespoon drained non-fat yogurt

1 teaspoon bee pollen (optional if allowed)

Method

1. Chuck it all in a blender or bullet! Blend until it looks green and creamy.

TIP: If you want a crunchy texture and salty taste add finely chopped celery to your dish before adding dressing.

IMPORTANT: A non-fat yogurt allowance is only added after several weeks on Gerson Therapy and when recommended by your practitioner.

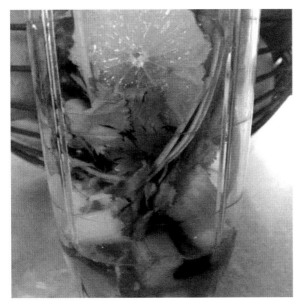

Before the blend!

Crunchy Creamy Green Sauce

If you've been craving crunchy and 'kinda' salty, try this. Great over a baked potato or as a dressing over your salad.

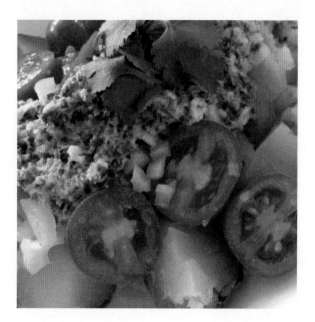

You'll need:

½ cup non-fat yogurt

2 teaspoons flaxseed oil

Bunch of parsley

Garlic (optional)

2 stalks celery

Method

1. Place everything except celery into a blender. Blend until green and smooth.

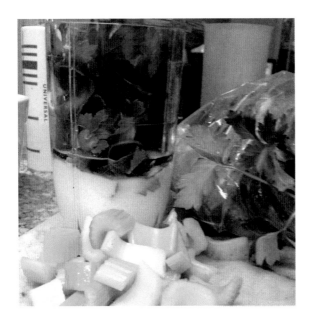

2. Add celery stalks (roughly chopped) and blend again only for a short burst. This gets the salty (celery is high in sodium) into the sauce but leaves 'bits' of celery still to provide crunch and texture.

TIP: Add extra celery finely diced for extra crunch.

IMPORTANT: A non-fat yogurt allowance is only added after several weeks on Gerson Therapy and when recommended by your practitioner.

Creamy Corn Sauce (Faux Cheese Sauce)

Close your eyes and it might taste and feel like cheese in your mouth! Serve over cooked vegetables or baked potato.

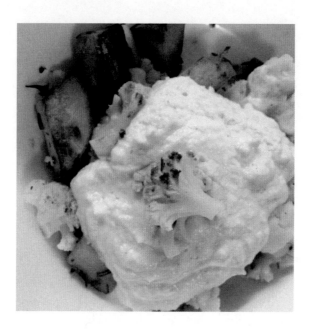

You'll need:
Corn kernels from 1 cob (raw)
About 1/2 cup cauliflower (cooked)
1 teaspoon honey
1 tablespoon flaxseed oil

Method:

1. Blend raw corn and cooked cauliflower with honey until smooth.
2. With blender running, drizzle in flaxseed oil to create creamy texture.

Rosemary Orange Dressing

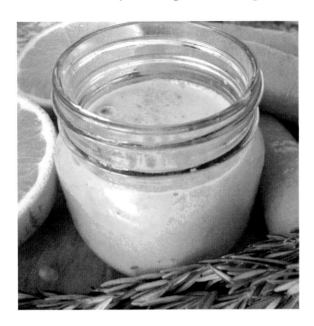

You'll need:

Juice of one carrot

1 orange, peeled and chopped (remove seeds)

1 teaspoon fresh Rosemary (or to taste)

2 teaspoons flaxseed oil

Garlic (optional)

Method

1. Place all ingredients into a blender or bullet.

GT Dressing

This is my staple Gerson Therapy dressing. Also try using lime juice without the honey.

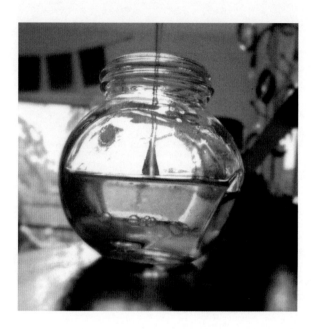

You'll need:
Equal amounts of:
Flaxseed oil
Lemon juice
Raw honey

Method

1. Shake to emulsify.

TIP: I keep mine in fridge for several days.

Grapefruit Dressing

If you like grapefruit, you've got to try this dressing! Goes very well with a salad of arugula (also known as rocket), tomatoes, roasted pumpkin, carrot and pear.

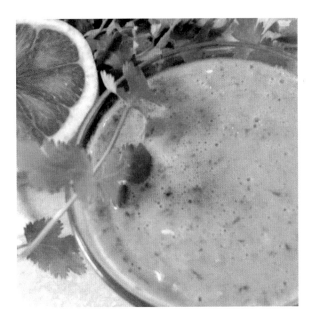

You'll need;
Grapefruit (ruby or yellow)
Bunch of cilantro
Teaspoon flaxseed oil

Method

1. Place all ingredients in blender or bullet and blend until smooth.

Thai Dressing

For an easy meal add a handful of salad on top of a baked potato and pour this over.

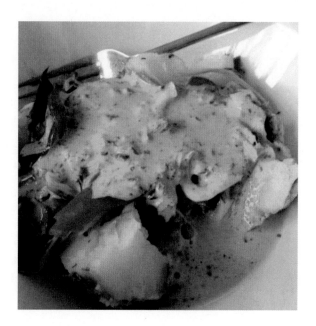

You'll need:
Non-fat yogurt
Coriander (cilantro)
Flaxseed oil
Juice of a lime

Method

1. Place all ingredients into a blender (or bullet) and blend until smooth.

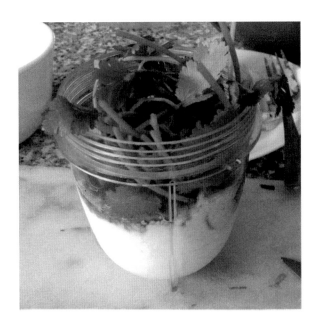

IMPORTANT: A non-fat yogurt allowance is only added after several weeks on Gerson Therapy and when recommended by your practitioner.

Tangy Horseradish Dressing

Recipe by *Tori Purple*

This dressing has a tiny kick and thick enough to be like mayonnaise.

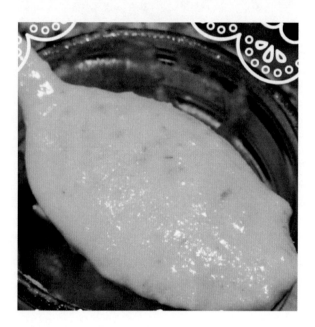

You'll need;

1/4 cup lemon juice

1/3 cup apple cider vinegar

1/4 cup flax oil

1 clove garlic

1 inch horseradish root - more if you want more spice

1 medium cooked cold potato

Fresh herbs (like dill and cilantro)

Method

1. Blend all ingredients together.

Orange Creamy Corn Dressing

This raw quick dressing is creamy. So creamy you'd think there is dairy in it! But there's not. It's delicious with hot or cold potatoes.

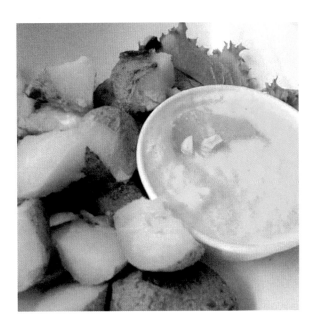

You'll need;

1 orange

1 corn cob

1 teaspoon flaxseed oil

Method

1. Remove rind and seeds from orange. Chop.
2. Cut kernels off cob.
3. Blend corn, flaxseed oil and 3/4 of orange pieces.
4. Once blended add extra orange pieces for citrusy surprises.

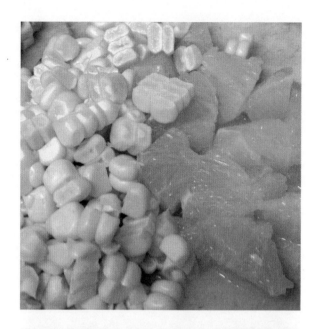

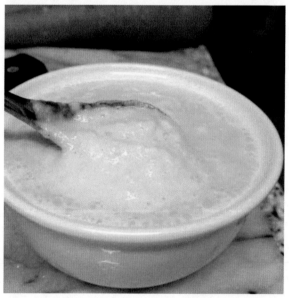

DRINKS

Champagne "Gerson" Vintage

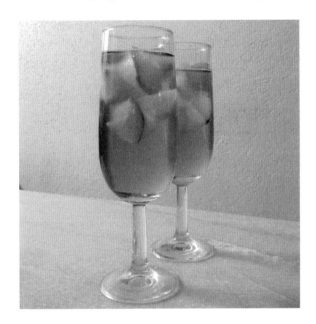

You'll need:

3 organic peppermint teabags

Dash of Essiac (optional)

Lemon/lime ice cubes

2 cups distilled water

Method

1. Add hot water to teabags and leave to cool. Tea bags can stay in.
2. Place a few lemon/lime ice cubes into a champagne flute.
3. Gently pour iced tea in over ice cubes.
4. Add a dash of Essiac.

Gerson Power Smoothie

If you cannot take another day of porridge for brekkie try this...

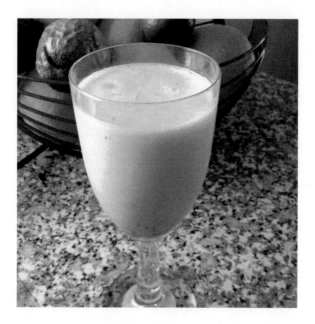

You'll need;

Non-fat yogurt

Flaxseed oil

Passionfruit (you could use any fruit)

Ice cubes (made with distilled water)

Cooked oats

Method

1. Place all ingredients into a bullet mixer or blender and blend until smooth.

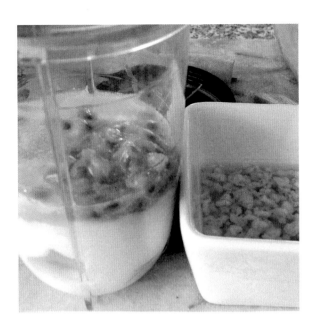

TIP: Make sure your oatmeal is cooked with plenty of water. But if it's too thick you could add a bit of water.

IMPORTANT: A non-fat yogurt allowance is only added after several weeks on Gerson Therapy and when recommended by your practitioner.

Lemon Lime Ice Blocks

Eat as is as a cool treat to suck on or add to iced peppermint tea. Serve in a long tall glass and you'll feel like you're at a holiday resort sipping a cocktail! A cocktail that is healing you!

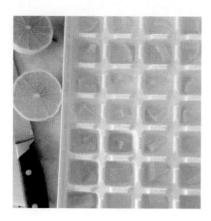

You'll need:

Segments of lemon or lime

Distilled water

Method

1. In an ice tray add tiny segments of lemon or lime.
2. Cover with distilled water and freeze.

TIP: Experiment with other fruits such as passionfruit.

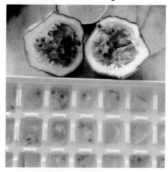

Pau D'Arco Tea

This isn't really a tea but a traditional antifungal bark which is allowed on the protocol. Its subtle flavor is delightful … hot or cold.

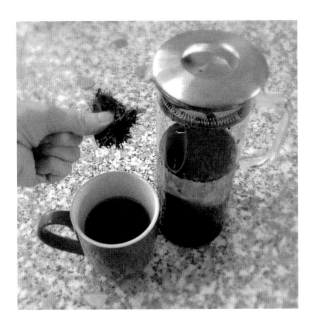

You'll need:
Pau D'Arco Tea
Distilled water

Method

1. Seep for 20 minutes. The longer the better.

TREATS

Baked Apple Dessert

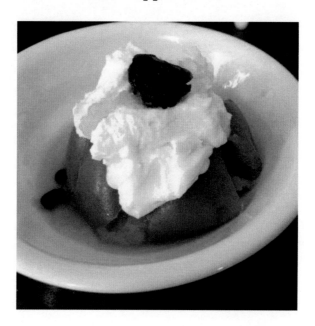

You'll need;

2 green apples

1 tablespoon dried fruit (currants and dates were used in the photo)

Drained non-fat yogurt to serve (if allowed)

Method

1. Core apples with an apple corer but do not peel. Slice bottom off so they sit flat in a small oven proof pan (with a lid).
2. Fill core holes with the dried fruit and cover.
3. Cook for 30 minutes in oven at 300°F (150°C).
4. Serve with drained non-fat yogurt if allowed.

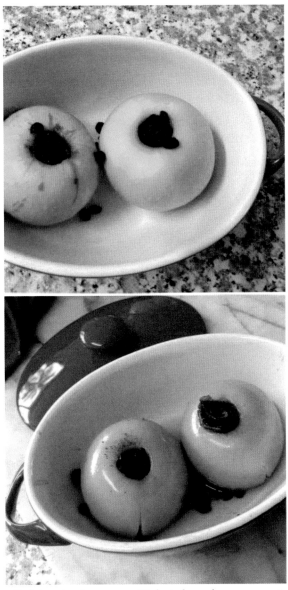

Left is going into oven. Right is how they came out!

Baked Banana-Peach Pancakes

Recipe by *Jfur Simpson*

Don't be fooled by the long description. This recipe is really quick and simple. A few dry ingredients. A couple of wet ones. Mix together, plop on sheet, set timer, done.

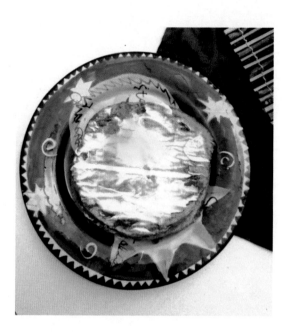

You'll need;

1 cup oat flour (easily made using the Norwalk "flour grid" and organic rolled oats, or a coffee grinder, flour mill, etc)

1 tsp (GT approved) featherweight Baking Powder (sodium/gluten free optional)

1 medium peach (or apple or other fruit of choice. Experiment!)

1 ripe banana (or apple)

1 sprinkling of allspice

Method

(Norwalk Juicer Method):

1. Preheat oven to 350°F (180°C) and place parchment paper on cookie sheet/baking tray.
2. Mix dry ingredients in bowl small enough to place under Norwalk shoot.
3. Using largest grid, place banana and quartered peach in Norwalk shoot, mashing down with the pusher so they fit. Be sure to have pusher in shoot BEFORE TURNING ON MACHINE or you will quickly have a banana-peach ceiling (BPC). Run banana and peach thru Norwalk and mix mush into dry ingredients adding a little distilled water to reach desired consistency.
4. Pour or scoop mixture onto cookie sheet and flatten/form into "pancakes" with spoon. (Can also lay second sheet of paper on top if you want the final pancake to be flat on both sides, and turn over have way through baking time. I don't bother anymore)
5. Bake 350°F (180°C) for 15-20 min (adjust for your oven and taste)
6. Spread finished pancakes with thickened (drained) organic non-fat yogurt and your daily allotment of organic maple syrup/raw honey. DEVOUR (I mean, enjoy!)

- Cooking pancakes in oven gives more consistent results than in a pan on stove and you can do them all at once, don't have to stand in front of the stove.
- If you don't have a Norwalk, you can still make the flour with a coffee grinder, food processor, or flour mill, and the smashed banana/peaches can be processed in a blender, food processor, hand mixer, potato masher, fork, etc.
- **IMPORTANT:** A non-fat yogurt allowance is only added after several weeks on Gerson Therapy and when recommended by your practitioner.

Gerson Custard

Who knew mixing non-fat yogurt with flaxseed oil creates a creamy custard texture. If you want it sweeter add your honey or sugar allowance.

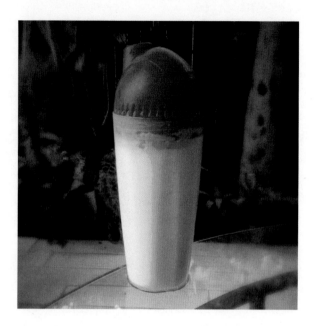

You'll need;

2 cups non-fat yogurt

2-4 tablespoons of flaxseed oil

Method

1. Into a 'shake' container (for quick easy pouring once done) add non-fat yogurt first. Then flaxseed oil and shake.

IMPORTANT: A non-fat yogurt allowance is only added after several weeks on Gerson Therapy and when recommended by your practitioner.

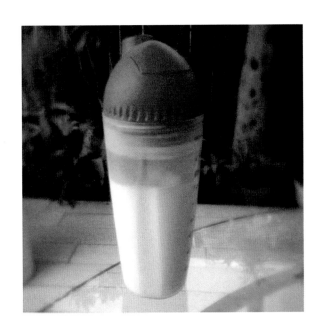

Chocolate-less Thick Shake

Recipe by *Nina Lesnanska*

August is a great time of year in Australia for us Gerson persons as black sapote aka chocolate pudding fruit is season!

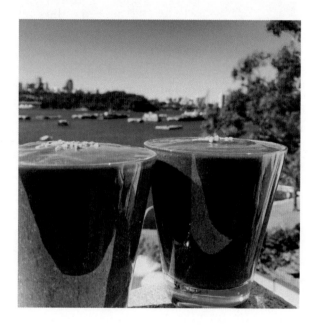

You'll need;

1 black sapote

1/2 small papaya

3/4 banana

2 cups of gruel (with oats not strained out)

1 teaspoon of bee pollen

A tiny dash of maple syrup

Method

1. Mix in a Vitamix or blender.
2. Sprinkle with bee pollen to serve. NB: view not included!

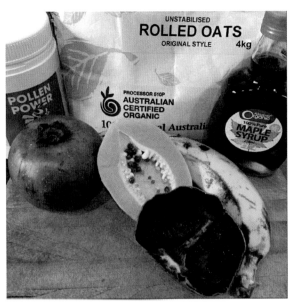

If you can't get black sapotes, leave it out for a yummy fruit thick shake.

Cream and Feta

Make a deliciously thick cream from non-fat yogurt by draining it but … only if non-fat yogurt has been recommended by your practitioner.

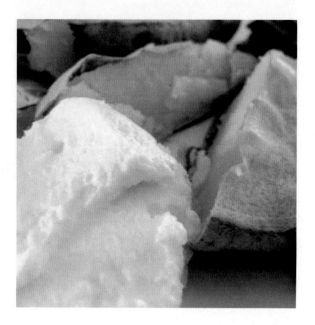

You'll need;

Non-fat yogurt (organic of course)

IMPORTANT: A non-fat yogurt allowance is only added after several weeks on Gerson Therapy and when recommended by your practitioner.

Method

1. Put a cheese cloth (or clean dish/tea towel) over a bowl and secure with rubber band.

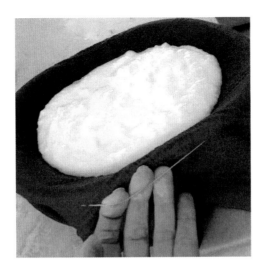

2. Pour non-fat yogurt on top of cloth. The liquid whey drains through. What's left on top of cloth is just like thick cream.
3. Leave drain in refrigerator.
4. The longer you leave it the thicker it gets. Leave it overnight and you will get a feta cheese texture which is fabulous in salads.

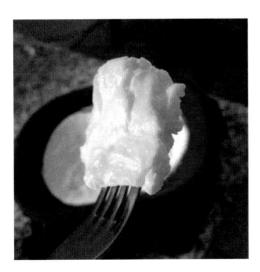

Cherry Orange Parfait

This was my dessert on Christmas Day. Yummo.

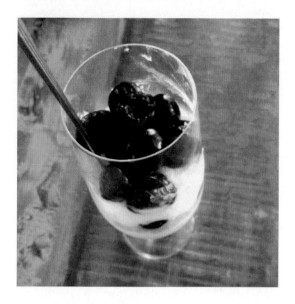

You'll need;

1 orange

Pinch of allspice

Cherries

1 cup quark or drained non-fat yogurt

Method

1. Peel and seed orange. Chop into small pieces.
2. Mix orange with allspice into quark and refrigerate overnight (this intensifies flavors).
3. Spoon quark mixture into a tall glass alternating with pitted halved cherries.

IMPORTANT: A non-fat yogurt allowance is only added after several weeks on Gerson Therapy and when recommended by your practitioner.

Caramel Baked Banana

A treat for winter nights. Baking brings out the natural sugars in the fruit and makes a caramel like syrup while making the flesh chewy.

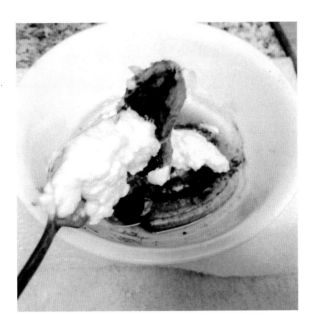

You'll need;
1 banana
Generous pinch of allspice
Drained non-fat yogurt to serve (if allowed)

Method

1. Slice banana length wise and place in shallow oven proof dish. (Most cereal bowls are oven proof so cook and serve in same dish.)
2. Sprinkle with allspice.
3. Bake uncovered 30 minutes at 350°F (180°C). Serve with a dollop of drained non-fat yogurt (if allowed) and another sprinkle of allspice.

Chard Chips

The drying concentrates the natural sodium. Probably only tastes salty to us peeps who now have a more sensitive taste sense. (Chard is also known as silverbeet)

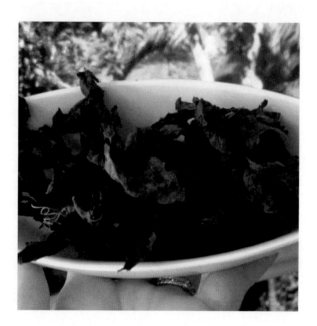

You'll need;

Chard

Method

1. Remove stalks from chard.
2. Place in a low oven until crisp and crunchy and ... salty.

"Girthday" Cake

This is ideal for special occasions like birthdays so even the Gerson person can have a treat. Also known as GERSON APPLE SPICE CAKE from "The Gerson Handbook".

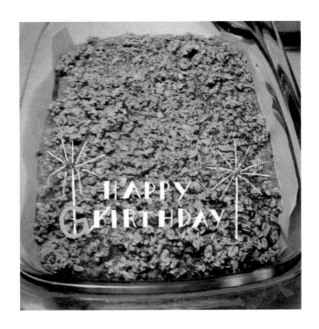

You'll need;

1/4 cup honey or maple syrup

1 cup fresh applesauce

1 ½ cups oat flour

3/4 cup whole wheat flour or triticale flour

3/4 cup crude brown sugar

Pinch allspice

Pinch mace

1/4 teaspoon ground coriander

2 cups raisins or chopped dates

1 teaspoon featherweight sodium free baking powder (optional) This is a potassium based baking powder. If you are a cancer patient, check with your physician first.

Crumb Topping;
2/3 cup rolled oats
1/3 cup maple syrup or honey
Pinch allspice
Pinch mace

Method

1. Combine wet and sifted dry ingredients.
2. Then add raisins or chopped dates
3. Pour into oblong baking pan lined with baking paper or dusted with rolled oats/flour.
4. To make topping, buzz oats briefly in blender to make a finer blend. Mix spices with oats. Mix in enough sweetener to make a crumbly mixture.
5. Sprinkle crumb topping on top.
6. Bake at 325°F (160°C) degrees for 40 minutes or until cake tests done (until a knife comes out clean).
7. Serve with a spoonful of fresh applesauce or non-fat yogurt (if allowed). ENJOY!

Oat Slice

Recipe by *Shelley Food Angel*

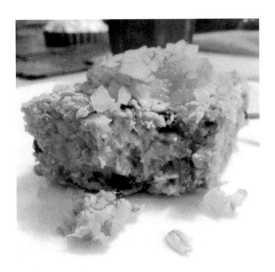

You'll need:

3 cups of pumpkin (cooked and mashed)

2 mashed bananas

3 cups rolled oats

1 cup oat bran

½ cup maple syrup

½ sultanas or soaked currants

Method

1. Mix all ingredients together.
2. Put into a baking dish lined with rolled oats to stop it sticking to the dish (or baking paper).
3. Bake for 1 hour at 300°F (150 °C).
4. Serve with chopped stewed apple and non-fat yogurt (if allowed).

NOTE: These are really heavy and very filling.

Popcorn

Hey it's not going to actually taste like popcorn but when sitting on the couch watching a movie with your family it just might! Ask nicely at your local cinema and they might give you some popcorn buckets for authenticity!

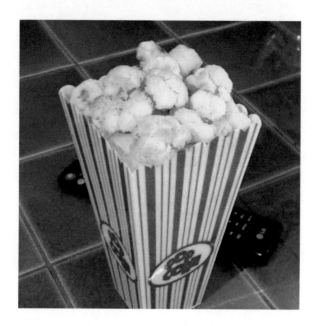

You'll need;
Cauliflower

Method

1. Break cauliflower into bite size bits.
2. Bake on baking paper at 30 minutes in oven set to 300°F (150°C) or until cooked.
3. Pop under grill to brown off at last minute.

Potato Puffs

Recipe by *Betsy Gahn*

This is my favorite way to eat potatoes as a treat during holidays and special occasions. They are nice salad with summer veggies and a dipping sauce! What's not to love! Yum!

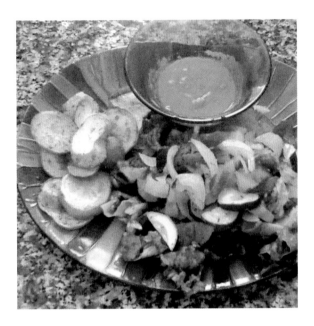

You'll need;
Potatoes

Method

1. Slice potatoes 1/4 inch or thinner.
2. Cook in single layer on cookie sheet or baking tray at 350-400°F (175 – 200°C) until browned and puffed.

Scones and Cream

Try this as a yummy alternative to porridge for breakfast or as a treat.

You'll need;
Oats
Apples
Non-fat yogurt
Honey (optional)
Allspice (optional)

Method

1. Slow cook oats and apple halves. Scoop out the cooked apple (eat separately or save for apple sauce).
2. Fill apples with cooked oats and top it with drained non-fat yogurt.
3. Add a drizzle of honey if you want it sweeter and a sprinkle of allspice if you want.

IMPORTANT: A non-fat yogurt allowance is only added after several weeks on Gerson Therapy and when recommended by your practitioner.

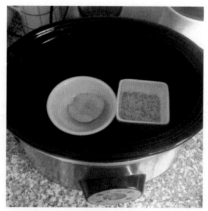

Cook the apple half and oats in a slow cooker in their serving dishes.(This doesn't work with all slow cookers as it seems to depend on the heat settings).

Smashed Banana Oat Cookies

Recipe by *Jfur Simpson*

The beauty of these cookies is in their simplicity. I can also eat them guilt free as my breakfast! But … this is a "complicated" recipe so pay CLOSE attention…

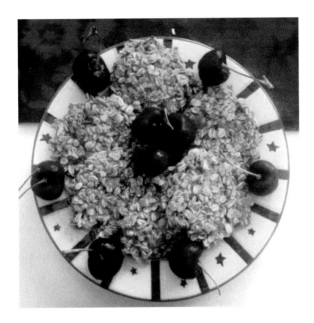

You'll need;
1 cup organic rolled oats

1 banana

Method

1. Put 1 cup organic rolled oats in a bowl.
2. Add banana in the bowl and smash it all together!
   *(Norwalk users: Put bowl of oats under shoot. Stuff banana in shoot. Put pusher in shoot <Do NOT, I repeat, DO NOT forget this step>. Turn on machine. Count "one thousand and…" DONE!)

3. Drop mixture in spoonfuls on cookie sheet/baking tray lined with parchment/baking paper. Bake at 350°F (180 °C) for 15-20 minutes.

YOU'RE DONE! OK… NOT SO FAST!

"What if I don't have parchment paper?" you ask.
Easy, lay rolled oats or oat flour on the sheet/tray instead. But I suggest you run, not walk, to Amazon… (Amazon.com)… NOT "The Amazon"….that would just be silly… and get yourself some. You will thank me for it. Look for the biggest roll and make sure it's unbleached.

"What if I can't have or don't like bananas?" Use apples, peaches, pears, a combo of all of the above. Mangoes would be out of this world! Juicy fruit will make them more moist. I use a combo of both apple and banana and add a touch of allspice. Harder fruit of course is harder to "Smash" so you may need a blender (or my personal favorite … a hammer!) if not using the Norwalk.

"Even with all that fruit they are still not sweet enough," I hear you say. Add your daily allotment of honey, maple syrup, unrefined sugar, etc. Also try adding reconstituted (plumped up in water) raisins.

Sourdough Potato Rye Bread

Cooked by *Nina Lesnanska*

This recipe is from the white Gerson Therapy book - page 369 for the bread recipe and page 366 for the sourdough starter. Nina peeled the potatoes - noting that the recipe doesn't say to peel or not. Nina says it was pretty easy to make for someone that has minimal baking experience.

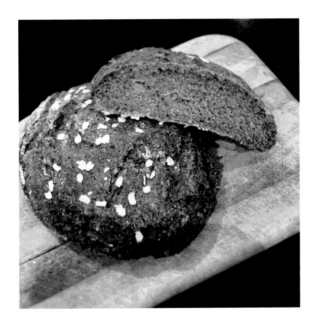

You'll need;

1 cup sourdough starter

2 cups warm mashed potato

1 1/3 cups potato cooking water

2 cups whole wheat or rye flour (Dr. Gerson allowed patients to use 1/3 wheat to 2/3 rye flour)

1/4 cup molasses (unsulphured)

1/3 teaspoon caraway or fennel seed

Method

1. Mix ingredients in a large non-metal bowl.
2. Cover and let stand in a warm place for several hours (or overnight for a very sour loaf).
3. Add the following: 1 1/2 to 3 cups rye flour as needed to make a workable dough.
4. Turn onto floured board and knead for 5-10 minutes.
5. Let dough rest for 5 minutes, then form into round or baton-shaped loaves.
6. Place on baking paper that has been well coated with raw oat flakes to prevent sticking.
7. Let bread rise until almost double (when bread does not spring back when lightly touched).
8. Bake at 350°F (180°C) for 50 minutes to 1 hour. For a very chew crust, place a pan of water in bottom of oven to create steam, or baste bread several times during baking with water. For soft crust, do not steam or baste.
9. Immediately wrap loaves in cotton towels after removing from oven. Let bread cool before cutting.

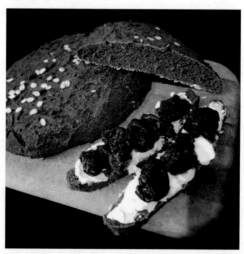

As a treat Nina serves the bread with non-fat quark and prunes!

Chapter 6: Random Tips & Time Saving Tricks

"The road less travelled is overrated; take the path of least resistance."
Helen Bairstow

Lost In Translation

Globally words can mean different things in the English language and I'd hate to think Gerson persons miss out on something allowed because it was called a different name!

- Anise aka aniseed
- Coriander aka cilantro
- Rocket aka arugula
- Silverbeet aka chard
- Courgette aka zucchini
- Eggplant aka aubergine
- Bell pepper aka capsicum
- Romaine lettuce aka cos lettuce

Juicer Hard Scum Cleaning Tip

Pam Holdsworth shared this…Does anyone get a build up of hard juice scum on the stainless steel juicer parts, despite washing them all the time? I have found an easy, chemical-free way to remove this without resorting to heavy scrubbing.

At the end of the day (or anytime when you wont be using your juicer for an hour or two) wash and rinse parts as normal, then while still wet sprinkle thickly with bi-carb of soda (sodium bicarbonate). This layer must cover all of the scum thickly. Then mist with vinegar until the bi-carb is saturated and starts to bubble and foam, but not too much to wash it off. (I have one of those cheap atomizers full of vinegar under my sink for lots of cleaning jobs). Let stand for at least one hour (or overnight) then scrub lightly, I find an old toothbrush or small bottle brush is good for this. If any stubborn scum remains, a light scrub with a plastic scourer should finish it off, or just repeat the bi-carb/vinegar process.

Cool Time Saving Tip From Jfur Simpson

Here's a cool technique (that only took me 2 yrs to discover): Freeze the entire green juice left-over fiber patty IN THE CLOTH. When it's frozen, it comes out in one piece, saving the need for bamboo liners or lots of scrubbing. You can clean the cloth as needed after emptying. This requires you have a few cloths, one to juice, one to freeze.

Things You 'Gotta' Have

We asked the Gerson Therapy Support Group what were things that you 'must' have while doing Gerson Therapy. Not the obvious like a juicer, but the little things…

Jfur Simpson said…

- Spiralizer (veggie noodle maker)

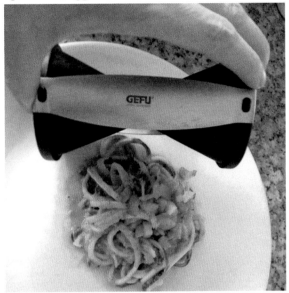

- Fresh herbs to compensate for salt withdrawal
- Stainless steel tongs
- oven mitts, or the willingness to put up with burns on your hands
- A personal shopper or a wheelie cart to haul your produce from the car
- Industrial sized bundles of paper towels
- A funnel
- A blender, mixer, magic bullet, etc
- Rubber gloves
- A step ladder to reach the ceiling splatters (Norwalk owners)
- Gallons and gallons of vinegar
- Aloe Vera plant
- A strainer

Pauline Perkins said…

- Green vegetable bags for longer lasting storage

- A decent mouli for the Hippocrates Soup! We started off with a little one but it took ages and gave me a sore neck, and so we invested in a large one and it's so much faster and easier!
- Lots of parsley - even grow your own!
- A compost bin

Rosette Husbands said…

- 8 oz canning jars to store carrot/apple juice for the day (if you can't make it fresh each time due)
- 24 oz canning jars to store soup and washed vegies for green juice
- Apple corer
- Salad spinner
- Sharp kitchen knife to chop big carrots and other fruits and vegies

Kathleen Blake said…

- Dr. Gerson's book "*A Cancer Therapy: Results of Fifty Cases*" to read while doing one's coffee break. This way the Gerson patient can read his very scientific, brilliant explanations for every part of his remarkable therapy and at the same time feel a connection to him and his love for humanity. (Available from Gerson.org)

Krista Clifton Adkins said…

- Brown towels, brown wash cloths and brown shirts!

Leanna Little Prosser said…

- Parchment or baking paper

- Gerson reference materials, especially *"Healing The Gerson Way"* by Charlotte Gerson
- A 2nd fridge!
- Storage containers for food (glass, stainless)
- A food scrubbing brush
- A lemon juicer (hand held)
- Lots of hydrogen peroxide
- A tiny pan for re-heating a single serving of Hippocrates soup
- Kitchen timers

Sup Box

This made life so much easier ... Look for craft or fishing tackle boxes. Make sure the lid seals the compartments so when it is closed and tips on side they don't all mix up. This box does make it easier as I don't have to unscrew and screw up all those bottles each time.

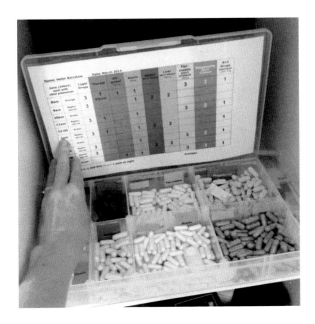

And if you get a larger box, A4 size, you can stick a laminated sup schedule to lid which can also double as a tick off chart using a white-board marker.

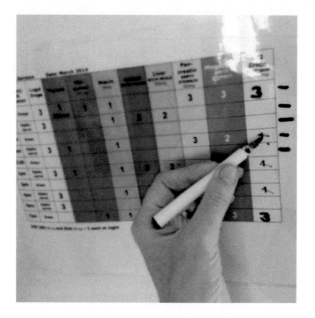

Useful Gerson Therapy Numbers

- **Cooked Oats**

  water:oats 3:1 (2:1 if you like it creamier)

  To cook oats, for every one part oats add three parts distilled water.

  E.g. for 4oz oats add 12oz water.

- **Coffee Concentrate** (4 full strength enemas)

  3/4 cup organic coffee (12 tablespoons) to 4 cups water.

  Boil 3 minutes uncovered and simmer for 15 minutes covered.

More Random Tips

Rather than heat coffee on the stove, I pour 8oz cold coffee concentrate (from jug in refrigerator) in the enema bucket (mine has measurements on side so this is very easy). Then add 8oz boiling and 16oz room temperature filterer/distilled water. Seems to equal the right temperature. If the coffee concentrate is room temperature you'll need much less hot water. And if I've only just made the coffee concentrate (i.e. it is hot) I don't need hot water. BTW a great tip is to get some good pouring jugs that hold about a litre (32oz). Seems we always need them.

Girls Will Be Girls

Here's a tip for the girls. Because us Gerson Persons use minimal skin and hair goop, you will save heaps of money. So ... spend a bit extra on a great 'style' cut. Pre-wash your hair before you go to the salon or take your own organic shampoo. And get a blow dry! (No toxins in hot air! And no styling product of course) Sounds vain but gee it makes you feel good.

Potassium Tip

You need to add this to every juice so store it in a bottle with a handy pourer (usually used for vinegar/oil) right next to your juicer. And if you're wondering what potassium is for, read "Healing The Gerson Way" by Charlotte Gerson which will explain the whole protocol.

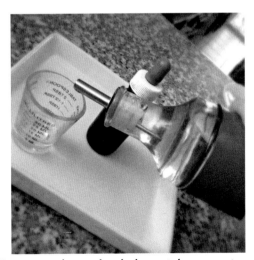

Put your iodine or lugols drops right next to it too.

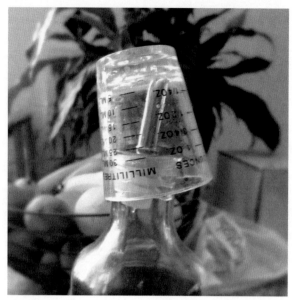

Store the measuring cup on top then you always know where it is!

Bee Pollen Sprinkles

Here's a storage tip that also makes for ease of use. Store your bee pollen in a sugar shaker in fridge for quick easy sprinkling.

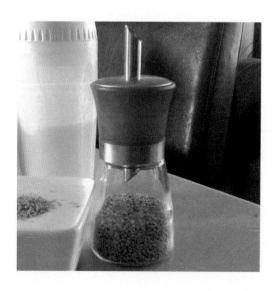

NOTE: Bee pollen can only added after several weeks on Gerson Therapy and when recommended by your practitioner.

Gerson Therapy Acronyms

CE = coffee enema

ACV = apple cider vinegar

MGT = modified Gerson Therapy

HTGW = Healing The Gerson Way (book by Charlotte Gerson available at Gerson.org or Amazon)

GT = Gerson Therapy

FGT = Full Gerson Therapy

NF = non fat

GI = Gerson Institute

GD = Gerson Doctor

NP = Naturopathic Doctor

CAJ = Carrot Apple Juice

CO = Castor Oil

COE = Castor Oil Enema

HR = Healing Reaction

GC = Gerson Coach

METS = metastasis (singular) or metastases (plural)

H2O2 = Hydrogen peroxide

And some creative (and hilarious) ones from people who have experienced Gerson Therapy first-hand and long term...

BS = Burning Sphincter (from COE!)

HAGMPTD = Having a Gerson meltdown. Prepare to duck.

COTC = Carrots on the ceiling! (From the Norwalk, not the meltdown).

...thanks Jfur Simpson

BO = Blow Out (from CE or Norwalk), alternatively it could just be for Body Odor (from not showering often because you don't have time, or a fluoride free water supply!)

...thanks Nina Lesnanska

YGPTCW? = You're Gonna Put That Coffee Where?
BPHSOMGNA = Baked Potato, Hippocrates Soup, OMG Not Again

...thanks Betsy Geist

KGTYH = Keep Going 'Till You're Healthy

...thank you Heather Thompson Scar

Two Coffee Questions

Penny Urich-Brenner explains two coffee FAQs with this excellent graphic...

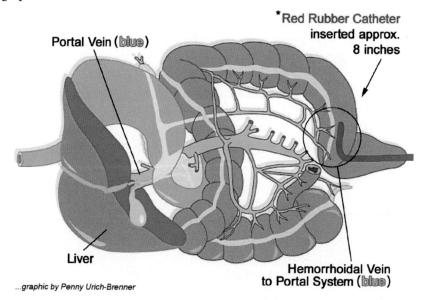

...graphic by Penny Urich-Brenner

Why lie on your right side?

This allows gravity to do its job. The veins (in blue) are on the right side of the colon. This position facilitates the components of the coffee that help in producing more bile and bile flow getting to the liver quickly: caffeine, palmitates, theobromine and theophylline.

Why is it necessary to insert the catheter 6-8 inches?

The distance from the anus over the second sphincter (bump) where the haemorrhoidal vein is located 5-6 inches. It's important to get past the second sphincter so the coffee absorbs into the vein system, which begins past that point. NOTE: It is very important to use the soft, pliable red rubber catheter, not the hard plastic tube that comes with the enema bucket, to avoid damage to the colon.

Chapter 7: Daring to Dream

"Stay close to Nature and her eternal laws will protect you."
Dr. Max Gerson

I wrote this back in May 2014 …
"Five months into my Gerson Therapy there are two things I want to say…

1. it went SO fast and I am actually looking forward to the next 19 months on the therapy.

2. sometimes it's useful to look back to acknowledge how far we've come… because I remember back in the first few weeks crying because I was so overwhelmed with all the rules, data and restrictions that Gerson Therapy imposes. I was so down that I felt like I'd rather die than live this way. I don't share this lightly. I'm sharing it because if you're new you might get an insight. I'm also sharing it because what got me 'up' and able to enjoy the therapy as much as I do now was … getting help! My fellow Gerson Persons with a 'huge' reason to heal, this is not a practice run. Beg borrow or do whatever you need. Ask. You HAVE to rest to heal. Might sound melodramatic but the alternative is not an option. For me, if I spend every cent healing, even go into debt, it's still a bargain!" *Helen Bairstow*

Thank you *Rachel Sharman* for your words of wisdom…
"I want to say something to those of you who are still in the midst of considering Gerson for healing and overall health. Listen, I know it is a big decision but I wish I had started the therapy sooner!!! I researched the Gerson Therapy almost 2 years before I was diagnosed with cancer. At that point I knew I would definitely do Gerson if I was ever diagnosed with

cancer. Why did I wait? Had realized that the issues I was having at that time (systemic Candida, menstrual issues, low thyroid, poor digestion, etc) were signs that something was wrong in my body, I would have acted immediately. They were precursors to my diagnosis of stage 3 uterine cancer at the age of 25 years old. I could have healed my body before cancer took hold. Before I had three little ones to care for. Before I had to deal with trauma of a cancer diagnosis. Please, if you look at the therapy and think "Well, that makes sense. That could work," then use that belief to propel you into health now instead of waiting for a cancer diagnosis or something more "life threatening". All disease comes from the same thing. It is all connected. Waiting may simply be giving your health more time to decline. Deficiency and toxicity are the two causes of every disease. You can deal with those two things right now. The Gerson Therapy does not claim to be a preventative therapy for those who are fully healthy, but who is fully healthy these days? You can use the principles of the therapy or the non-malignant protocol for many health issues. Do not look back in two years and wish you had been proactive. I am not trying to be preachy or get on my high horse. I am just telling you, one health seeker to the next, to act now - you will never regret it."

Tami Hadley McVay celebrates "The end" … or is it the "beginning"?
Just finished up my appointment with my Gerson Doc … I am officially off the full Gerson Therapy. Will be on maintenance now … 4 juices and 1 coffee break. Not exactly sure what to do with myself? No scheduled meals, juices, coffee breaks, supplements or sinkfuls of produce to wash? Kind of makes me anxious. This will be a bit of a transition to let go of my timer and spreadsheet. I have learned so much about loving myself these past 2 years. That's what Gerson Therapy is … the ultimate self-care. Giving yourself the utmost attention and care through nutritious food, juices, coffee breaks and supplements, so that the body can heal at its highest potential. Thank you Gerson Therapy for EVERYTHING! Perhaps I will celebrate with a 32oz bucket of coffee! Cheers!

This was posted by the amazingly awesome *Kathleen Blake* and it is a great way to finish this book …

"Twenty years from now you will be more disappointed by the things that you didn't do than by the ones you did do. So throw off the bowlines. Sail away from the safe harbor. Catch the trade winds in your sails. Explore. Dream. Discover." Mark Twain